To your continued
health and success!

Greg McEly

World Class Smiles:
The Consumer's Guide to Dental Implants
and Cosmetic Dentistry

TABLE OF CONTENTS

FOREWORD
Transform Your Smile Today!

Dr. Gregory McElroy is a leading authority in dental implant surgery in Encinitas, CA. He has been changing lives for over 25 years. Dr. McElroy's unparalleled position as a national dental authority is the result of numerous factors, including the following:

- Bestowed the status of Diplomat from the International Dental Implant Association (Their highest level of achievement awarded.)
- Placed among the top 1% of dentists with an authority in IV Oral Conscious Sedation
- One of the first to become certified in IV Oral Conscious Sedation
- Has trained over 200 dentists throughout his career
- Has managed over 25 dental offices in California and Arizona
- Has owned and operated three dental practices in San Diego County
- Trusted industry leader.

Dr. McElroy graduated from California State University Fullerton with a degree in Biology, and he earned his Doctor of Dental Surgery degree at Georgetown University in Washington, DC.

Aside from being one of the most trusted authorities in the industry, he possesses one of the most caring souls, believing wholeheartedly in giving back through charity and community service. Committed to improving lives around the globe, he plays an active, hands-on role in all sorts of charity work, including donating several thousand dollars per year to the Make a Wish Foundation of San Diego.

He has made three 4-day (12 hour workday) trips to the Dominican Republic in the last 5 years where he spent numerous hours performing advanced oral surgery, bone grafting, and dental implant placement to the tune of over $2,000,000 in free dental care. On one of those trips, he was accompanied by his son, Brandon, who assisted him and donated his time. On a separate trip, his son, Tyler, assisted and donated his time. Upon experiencing and helping in the many surgeries performed, Tyler was thrilled to offer his help as he took a liking to the incredible Dominican people. He decided at that time that he felt that same drive and motivation to do what his father does and applied to dental school.

Dr. McElroy and his team participate annually in Dentistry from The Heart, which provides free dental services to anyone in need in the local community. Dr. McElroy also donates regularly to the Wounded Warrior Project and sponsors local sports teams. The office participates in at lease one full day per year of charity events which are open to the public. They generally rotate between Dentistry from The Heart, which is open to all and Smiles For Freedom which is held around Veterans Day and is focused on veterans, members of the armed forces and first responders.

"Every good act is charity. A man's true wealth hereafter is the good that he does in this world to his fellows."
—Moliere

When Dr. McElroy was just 9 years old, he had a terrible dental phobia and bad teeth. Every single time he went to the dentist, it was a traumatic experience for him. He remembers telling his father, "Dad, I want to become a dentist." His father said, "Sure son, may I ask why you are choosing dentistry as a career?" Immediately upon being asked that question his answer was a resounding, "Because I think anyone could do a better job than that guy!" His sense of humor and motivation for a fulfilling career were created that day and never left him. As each year went by, his dream of becoming a dentist got closer and closer, and he worked hard to ensure that he was going to be the best he could be. Before he knew it, he awoke to find that he was the best dentist he could be, and dad could not be prouder.

 As the years went by and his practice thrived, he also raised a family. He looks forward to the day that he can pass the torch to one of his sons who has decided to follow in his footsteps.

When not working at the office, Dr. McElroy enjoys riding motorcycles, attending his four children's sporting events and spending time with his wife and family.

Dr. McElroy is a 5-star-rated dentist in Encinitas, CA, offering advanced dental care — serving Encinitas, Carlsbad, San Marcos, Vista, Oceanside, Solana Beach, Del Mar, Ranco Santa Fe, Escondido & San Diego, CA.

One of his favorite quotes:

"The harder I work, the luckier I get!"

Why is McElroy Smiles by Design Unique?

Practicing in Southern California, competition is fierce. This practice focuses on being customer centric. Every single member of the team is purely focused on putting the customers' needs before their own. Dr. McElroy understood from day one that it was important to make his business customer centered. He is in tune with and anticipates the needs of his patients, sometimes before they even know their needs themselves, and this mindset continues on through his team. Below are just a few ways they have strived to become unique in their customer service.

They Lead by Example

Leading by example is something Dr. McElroy and his team incorporate into the day-to-day. They also put up pictures of patients and allow them to share their experiences. By doing so, they learn how patients are affected by each and every part of their experience. This helps them to focus on what matters most.

They Embrace Patient Feedback

This practice believes wholeheartedly that feedback is a gift. Even behind the most negative feedback is a lesson to be better and an opportunity for the business to step up their game. Each team member takes the appropriate amount of time to listen to what their patients have to say, read customer comments, and tend to what needs to be done to make every patient 100% satisfied.

They Do Not Take Things at Face Value

It can be easy to get caught up in the daily grind, causing a business to lose sight of who they are there to serve. This is why Dr. McElroy takes the time to talk to and observe his patients, ensuring that he can get a better perspective on their thoughts. Where do they struggle? What are they thinking and feeling? Interacting with patients is what gives him a richer understanding of those he serves, helping him to gain new insights as to what they need.

They Work the Front Lines

Understanding what the patient needs cannot always be conveyed while they are sitting in the chair. This practice understands that sometimes they must step outside of their role and check out the front counter or take a customer call. This allows everyone involved to experience every aspect of a patient's needs and helps them to make awesome business decisions with the patient in mind. Taking in a patient's perspective changes a leader's view and opens up all sorts of opportunities to innovate the business!

In addition, the office has incorporated state-of-the-art technologies into the practice that makes their diagnosing abilities superior to most other dental practices. Dr. McElroy has created an environment where they are known as a one-stop-shop, allowing the patient the convenience of not having to travel to many different locations and providers to have their various advanced dental care needs met. He has created what he calls a "decision pyramid" that helps to answer any question he or a team member may have.

- ✔ What is best for the patient?
- ✔ What is best for the office as a whole to produce exceptional care?
- ✔ What is best for us, the individual?

If every question is first met by this decision pyramid, the answer can be found very quickly.

The #1 Reason This Dental Practice Gets Tons of Referrals – The Team!

People love the team – the staff, the doctors. In fact, Dr. McElroy describes his team as "the dream team". He states, without fail, that they are the best team in San Diego. He strives to always lead by example, and as a result, the upper tier of his team has been with the practice between 11 and 17 years. The doctors are friendly, knowledgeable, and caring. Not to mention the fact that patients are able to see the same doctor every visit and very rarely does any patient have to be referred out to a specialist.

The team is only as strong as its weakest link. A patient's experience starts the moment they first hear about this practice. The phone call must be perfect. Then they come to the office, and it is immaculate. To Dr. McElroy, every touch point must be perfect. The patient care rendered and follow up must be first class. At any time during this chain, if everything is not perfect the chain is broken and the relationship damaged. So, every point of contact is critical.

The Golden Rule - Treat Others How You Wish to be Treated!

Continuing Education

Dr. McElroy's dedication to continuing education has kept him up to date with the latest advances in dental medicine.

- Bestowed the status of Diplomat from the International Dental Implant Association (Their highest level of achievement awarded.)
- Awarded a Mastership from the International Dental Implant Association
- Awarded a Fellowship from the International Dental Implant Association
- Completed studies at the prestigious Las Vegas Institute for Advanced Dental Studies
- Studied nationwide with top clinicians, including Dr. Bill Dorfman of ABC's Extreme Makeover
- Earned his certification as a member and graduate of the Dental Organization for Conscious Sedation

Dr. McElroy is constantly studying and educating himself on the newest techniques and materials. He believes that most advances in dentistry and medicine are driven by technology, and while technology can be quite expensive, it is invaluable to the dedicated dental office.

The industry is ever changing. As advancements in technology continue to push us forward, Dr. McElroy believes that it is more important now than it ever has been before to stay up to date on the latest in preventative care and treatment. Continuing education has allowed him to become a master in not only dental implant surgery but also:

- Dental Cleanings
- Dentistry for Children
- Sedation Dentistry
- Teeth in a Day
- Dental Crowns
- Dental Bridges
- Root Canal Treatment
- Dentures
- Dental Bonding
- Veneers

- Teeth Whitening
- Emergency Dental Care
- Invisalign
- Teeth Straightening
- Wisdom Teeth
- Gum Treatment
- TMJ and Teeth Grinding
- Sleep Apnea Treatment
- Athletic Mouthguards
- Cosmetic Dentistry

By consistently continuing his education, Dr. McElroy and his team have become highly educated by the absolute best in their field, continually expanding their specialties and knowledge.

Mentorship

Choose a job you love, and you will never have to work a day in your life
- Confucius

Dr. McElroy has had many mentors over his years of service. In the early years, he gives credit to Dr. Robert Cadalso, and in the later years Dr. Arun Garg and the Scheduling Institutes, Jay Geier. He feels that he was fortunate to have worked for a large corporate dental operation early in his career. It was there that he was presented with the opportunity and pleasure of hiring and training hundreds of dentists in both California and Arizona. Mentorship has always been something he is proud to provide.

In addition, he has attended many Tony Robbins events and has learned much from his teachings. For those of you who may not know, Tony Robbins is a self-help coach who educates you to innovate, expand, be better, pursue your dreams and change your perception in order to succeed. He believes that everything has the meaning that you give it!

Some of the things Dr. McElroy has learned from Tony Robbins:

- How to articulate core values
- How to identify goals and define a vision for success
- How to create professional growth plans
- How to manage important business transactions
- How to identify limiting beliefs
- How to foster more powerful connections
- How to obtain a work/life balance
- How to communicate more succinctly and effectively

"There is a powerful driving force inside every human being that, once unleashed, can make any vision, dream, or desire a reality."
−Tony Robbins

The top three takeaways you will get from this practice:

✔   The best in customer service
✔   State-of-art beautiful facility
✔   One-stop-shop with advanced dental services

CHAPTER 1

Why Read This Boring Little Book?

Let's be honest, there are a heck of a lot more exciting things you could spend your time reading. You know that, I know that, and anyone who sees what you are reading knows that, too. It's not every day that people recommend a book about choosing a dentist. They don't hit the bestseller lists, and nobody is lined up to turn it into a movie. Having said all of that, there are still some really good reasons to read this boring little book.

When it comes to your family, you want what is best for them. But what you may not realize is that without nice teeth and a great smile they may not go as far in life. The truth of the matter is that those who have teeth problems tend to fall behind, be bullied, not be confident, and get lower grades. What child wants to stand in front of the classroom to speak when they have teeth that people laugh at? Helping your family get their best start in life includes making sure they have excellent dental care.

How much would you say you trust your dentist? Trust is a huge factor when it comes to your dentist. You need to trust that the person will suggest treatments that you really need, rather than ones that will simply line their pockets. Are you tired of walking out of the dental office with a big bill in your hand, and a huge question in your heart as to whether or not you really needed all that work to begin with? Having a dentist you trust is crucial to getting care that you will feel comfortable with.

Remember when you were a child and your parents took you to either the only dentist in town or they just grabbed one from the phone book? Nobody paid much attention to what dentist they went to, and most people didn't know why it mattered at all anyway. Well, guess what happened? It created a generation of people who feared the dentist, because they often had poor experiences. I'm here to tell you that today, you don't have to worry so much.

You can relax.

Today we realize how important it is to choose the right dentist. Not every dentist makes a good fit for every person, and vice versa. If you want to have the best possible experience, you have to take the time to learn about what makes a great dentist, how to go about choosing one, and what you can expect from them. That's where this book comes into play.

I've written this book to take the guesswork out of the equation. I know for the person reading this it can be confusing to choose a dentist. Do you choose one based off location? How about their experience and specialties? What about ones that are offering a coupon to get me in the door? These are all legitimate questions and they are often part of what goes into why people choose the dentist that they choose. But is answering these questions good enough? The short answer is no, there's more that needs to go into it.

Choosing the right dentist isn't rocket science, so don't worry that you will be spending a lot of time trying to figure this out. But once you finish reading this book, you will have a good sense of what makes for a good dentist, why choosing the right one should matter to you, and where to begin your search.

For many people, the right dentist may come along only once in a lifetime. When they move out of reach of that dentist, or if the dentist retires, the person may feel as though no other dentist can replace that person. That's how much you want to love your dentist. You want to feel like there's nobody who could replace that person, because they make you feel that they care about you as a patient, they have your best interest at heart, and they are one-of-a-kind in the field.

It's important to realize as well that a lot has changed over the years when it comes to dentistry. While you may have memories from your childhood of going to the dentist and it being scary, the technology has come a long way. Sit in the dentist's chair today and you will see all the high-tech equipment used to quickly get pictures of your teeth, fill cavities, and apply fluoride. You will be pleased to know that sitting in the dentist chair for 20 minutes with a bulky fluoride tray in your mouth, drool seeping out the sides, is a thing of the past. Today, fluoride is applied in a couple of minutes and the patient is on their way out the door, able to go about their business.

A lot has changed in dentistry over the years, making it a much more patient-friendly experience.

There are a lot of things that people worry about when it comes to choosing a dentist. They have their initial fears of the dentist, because they believe that there's going to be pain involved. A lot of pain. Then there are the fears about how much work will be needed, if the dentist is qualified to do all that is needed, and how much the bill is going to be. Then there are added fears about being able to schedule appointments around work or school, and other added stressors.

These are quite honestly issues that you don't have to worry about, and by the time you finish reading this book, my hope is that I've helped you to see that. Dentistry is quite painless today, because modern technology has helped to address that issue. Plus, nearly every dentist has a variety of payment options to help you be able to comfortably afford any treatment you may need. Your first priority should be to get the treatment that you need, not spend time worrying about paying for it. That is usually solved without any issues. Add to that the fact that many dentists today offer weekend and evening hours, and you can see that the fear of when you will be able to fit in an appointment is something you no longer need to worry about as well.

Many people put off going to the dentist because they fear costs, but what they don't realize is that actually works against them. The best thing you can do is to focus on prevention. When you can help prevent problems from arising, you will help to keep expenses down. Ignoring going to the dentist or getting treatment for something that needs to be done tends to increase the costs. Prevention is the first goal in the dental world. The second would be to have the necessary treatment right away, before it gets worse.

I've known numerous patients who started out needing to have a small cavity filled. They put it off, for whatever reason, thinking that by delaying the treatment they were putting off expenses and the work. The problem with this is that the cavity continues to get worse. Then you have a bigger cavity that needs to be filled, and the bigger the cavity, the more you are risking needing a crown, which will add a lot to the treatment expense.

Simply taking care of the issue at hand as soon as it's identified can help to keep costs down. Going to the dentist twice per year for your check-ups and cleanings can also help to keep expenses down, because it keeps your teeth in a healthier condition. Keeping plaque removed from teeth, through regular dental visit cleanings, can go a long way toward helping to keep your teeth and gums healthy for years.

The bottom line is that if you want to be able to smile and laugh without trying to cover your mouth up out of embarrassment. Well, that doesn't just happen on its own. You need to have a dentist you can trust who will help guide you, identify where there are issues and help you find the best treatment, and help you feel comfortable.

Why Choosing the Right Dentist is A Must

1. You and your family want to feel comfortable and confident every time you go to the dentist. You can only have that comfort if you know you have the right dentist for you.
2. Your smile is the first thing that most people notice about you. It's also the cornerstone of your confidence. Loving your smile is essential to feeling confident talking to people, laughing in front of others, and in loving what you see when you look in the mirror.
3. Having the right dentist for you means that you will always be able to get the appointments you need. You won't have to stress about how to fit them into your schedule or try to take off work or school to always get them done.
4. You will know that you have a dentist that keeps up with the changes in the industry and uses advanced technology in order to bring you the most comfortable experience.
5. You will know that the dentist you choose has a great reputation and is well respected. The dentist will have a track record of being great with other patients, helping you to feel more comfortable about what they can do for you and your family.
6. You want your kids to grow up feeling good about who they are and how they look, rather than having teeth that have problems that lead them to being bullied. You want to feel confident when you shake hands with someone in the office, and you want your kids to no longer be embarrassed when they get called to the front of the classroom to give a presentation.

We have all known someone who covers their mouth up when they laugh in a crowd. Or maybe they don't want to show their teeth when they smile. They may even be the child who hides in the back of the room, afraid to go before his peers because he doesn't like his teeth. Whether we realize it or not, how we feel about our teeth plays a major role in how we feel about ourselves as a whole.

Let's say that again another way, because it's so important that we understand it. How you feel about your teeth helps to lay the foundation for how you feel about yourself overall. It also helps others to form their opinion about you. While adults may be a bit kinder when it comes to someone who has problems with their teeth or smile, children are not. Let's be honest in saying that they can be absolutely brutal.

If you feel bad or embarrassed about how your teeth look or feel, then there's a good chance you will suffer. You won't want to smile, participate, laugh, or do many of the things we associate with happiness and being successful. Being happy with the teeth and smile you have makes a major difference in your life.

When you have teeth and a smile that you love and are comfortable with, you are more inclined to:

- Be happier with yourself and in life in general. When you love the way your teeth look, you will find yourself more able to smile and be happy.
- Speak up, speak out, and participate more. You will no longer be the adult hiding in the back of the boardroom or the child who hides in the back of the classroom, afraid of speaking in front of the group.
- Have more confidence in everything you do. People who love their teeth and smile will smile more, coming across as friendly. They may find that they speak to more people have more relationships as a result.

Being confident with your teeth makes you more confident in life, which helps you do more, achieve more, and have more fun. Aren't you tired of having to try and hide your smile or cover your mouth when you laugh? You don't have do these things anymore. It all comes down to finding the right dentist and putting your trust in the person to help you have the best teeth and smile going forward.

If you are like me, and like most other people in the country, you want to be happy. Smiling tends to make people happier, and being happier leads to being more positive. We can all use some more positivity in our lives. Research shows that when we smile more there are many things that take place, including everything from lowering your stress level and negative thinking patterns to increasing your attention span and productivity.

It may be hard to believe that so much is weighted on a smile, BUT IT REALLY IS. Our smile is not only something we notice about ourselves, but it's also one of the first impressions others have of us. And you know how important first impressions can be. A smile has a major impact on such things as getting hired for a job, being more easily remembered, others finding us attractive, and more. Most people conducting interviews know within the first seconds of meeting the person whether or not they are in the running for the position. The smile says it all. Flash a smile that has crooked, dull teeth that are filled with stains and plaque and you can kiss that job goodbye.

When you smile, your brain releases dopamine, serotonin, and endorphins, which are feel good neurotransmitters. They help to relieve stress and pain, and keep you feeling good and happy. These neurotransmitters help us to be more confident, and better able to cope in life. Smiles are also contagious, with people often unconsciously responding to a smile with a smile. As you can see, the importance of our smile goes beyond what you see in the mirror. There is science behind the importance of it and the role that it plays in our everyday lives.

A great smile is essential to a happy life in today's world.

A simple act of a smile can quite literally transform your world. And I'm not just saying that because I spend my life helping to create beautiful smiles. Loving your smile will help you want to show it more. When you

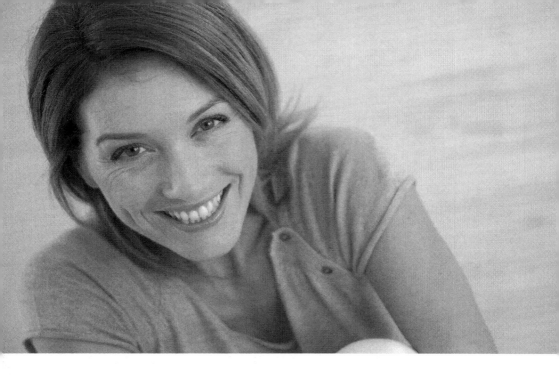

use the insider secrets to choose the right dentist for you, you will be on the right path to loving your smile. There's nothing quite like having beautiful teeth and healthy gums.

Choosing the best dentist for you and your family is an important role, and one that you want to put some effort into. Choosing the right one can make a huge difference when it comes to dreading your appointments or looking forward to them. It can also help set the stage for how your children grow up to feel about going to the dentist. The last thing you want is for your child to fear going to the dentist and to take that with them into adulthood.

When you choose the right dentist for you and your family, you will be confident in every visit. You will have someone that you trust is putting your best interest first and that they hear you, see you, and understand you not only as a patient, but as a person. I know I don't want to be just another number that gets called and serviced. I want to be with professionals who care that I'm there and see me as a person with fears, concerns, wishes, and plans.

So why read this boring little book? Because while it will help you find the right dentist for you and your family, it is going to do far more for your family beyond that.

CHAPTER 2

How to Confidently Choose the Best Dentist for Your Family

Did you know that finding the right dentist for you and your family is not just a cosmetic issue? It's a health issue as well. Misaligned, "crooked" teeth EQUAL significant medical problems. Poorly aligned teeth can produce chronic headaches and migraines, contribute to digestive problems because of poor chewing of foods, make getting a decent night's sleep impossible, and, maybe most dangerous, foster gum disease. Gum disease has absolute links to diabetes, heart disease, strokes and dementia, as well as, of course, loss of natural teeth altogether.

There is a lot riding on the importance of you finding the right dentist.

When you think about the number of dentists that there are to choose from, it's easy to see why it can be a daunting task to choose one. Well, not just one, but the right one. Anyone can choose a dentist, but not everyone will do some homework in order to choose the right dentist, and there's a huge difference between the two. Choosing the right dentist for your family is going to set your mind at ease. It's going to help your family to feel comfortable and confident as they go in for their appointments. And if the time arises that they need treatment, they won't run out the door or try to hide to keep it from happening.

There are over 160,000 dentists in the country. Open your local phone book or do a quick Google search and you will without a doubt find many that are in your local area. You have more dentists available to you than you could care to ever want or need. But don't let that overwhelm you. Choosing the right dentist comes down to one thing.

Confidence.

Confidence, by definition is having faith that you the choice you make will be the right one. I've talked with many parents over the years, and I hear how they fear making the wrong choice. Until they came to my office they lacked the confidence that it took to make a dentist selection based on something more than just choosing a name. You probably never gave it much thought, but choosing a dentist should be treated like you are hiring someone for a job. In essence, that's exactly what you are doing.

Time Well Spent

There isn't one thing you can do to choose the right dentist for your family. I wish it were that easy, as I'm sure you do as well. Rather, it's a variety of things that you will do in order to help lead you to the right selection. Don't worry, though, I don't want you to think this is a process that is going to be ultra time-intensive. You shouldn't have to spend a great deal of time on these things.

Going back to the health implications of making sure you have the right dentist, it goes further than you may realize. When teeth are not properly cared for, the gums can pull away from the teeth, which allows pockets and the harboring of infection. Periodontal disease turns into a VERY difficult, painful and costly problem later in life. Most people don't realize it, but the $4,000 that is not spent during the teen years can easily require a $40,000 full-mouth restoration later in life.

Not only that, but periodontal disease compromises health and often leads to tooth loss and the need for dentures. Gum disease is serious business. It increases the complications and risks of other diseases, such as diabetes, heart disease, strokes, and dementia.

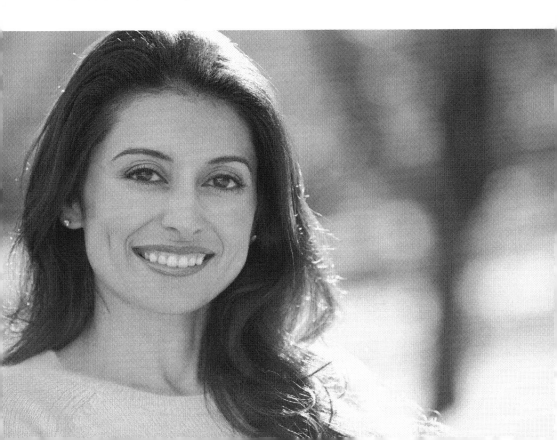

Yes, it will take some to find the right dentist. But it's going to be time well spent and it will be well worth it in the long run. It can help you and your family avoid many awful diseases, pain, and embarrassment, possibly even helping to avoid earlier death due to some of those diseases. Think about how much time you have spent choosing or going to a dentist who doesn't feel right for you. By putting in a little time to find the right one, you can help avoid the dreaded feeling you get when it's time for the next appointment. You will no longer be sitting in the waiting room wondering if you should have found another dentist prior to that appointment, and when will you ever finally get busy doing it?

The questions will be over, the doubt will be over, and you can stop wishing you had a better dentist, or one that is a better fit for your family. By putting in the time to read this book and doing a little of the legwork that is recommend in it, you will walk away with a dentist who is perfect for your family. In the whole scheme of things, that alone is going to save you a lot of time, headache, doubt, stress, and more.

While there are specific questions you will want to ask the dentists you interview for the job, and yes, that's what you are essentially doing, we will cover those in a later chapter. For now, let's look at some of the other things you can uncover and discover in order to help make you feel confident about choosing the right dentist for your family.

Remember, the time you put into finding the right dentist is an investment in your family's dental health, as well as their psychological well being and long term health and longevity. SO DON'T TAKE SHORT CUTS. We want to do what we need to in order to weed out those who are not a good fit and get to the best of the best. Keep in mind that the best of the best for someone else may not be the best of the best for your family. You may have different needs, wants, and goals, and you will need to keep that in mind as you go along.

Where to Look
There are many places to look to begin your search for the right dentist, but let's take a look at some of the most popular options. This way we can take a look at the pros and cons of these choices and narrow down which may be the better routes to consider taking.

You will find that advice and information regarding choosing a dentist abounds. But that doesn't mean you should listen to all of the advice you receive. As with anything else, you should consider the source, take some things with a grain of salt, and still take steps to include researching the candidate. There's nothing that will replace simply doing some good old-fashioned research on the person you are considering hiring as your family dentist.

Some of the most popular ways that people find new dentist leads include:

- Recommendations they may receive from their friends, family members, or co-workers.
- By conducting searches online and reviewing their website, social media pages, or reading reviews about them.
- Through general advertising that you may see online, on a billboard, in a magazine, or on the television.
- Seeing a dentist be featured in a news story, whether on television or in print, or in another type of article or news story.
- Spotting a dentist's office as you are driving near your home, school, or office.
- By looking at the in-network provider list provided by your insurance company.

There may be additional ways that people find their way to a dentist, but these are the most common ways. In order to find the right dentist for your family, you have to start out with knowing where to look for them. Once you have narrowed down a few ideal candidates, that is when you will be ready to move on to taking the step of researching and interviewing them.

Ideally, you will come up with a short list of candidates that you will take the time to evaluate. This is the most effective way to determine the best doctor for you. Sometimes people may look good on paper, but they have a personality that doesn't click with your family. Or perhaps they look a little sterile on paper and in looking at their credentials, but when you meet there is an instant connection with their personality. Their credentials matter a lot, but so too does their personality, so that they fit in well with your family and help you to feel comfortable and secure when you go in for every visit.

You want a dentist you not only feel comfortable with, but who you trust, and who you feel will listen to you and your family. Everyone wants to feel heard and that they are cared about, but many dentists are in such a hurry today that they limit their interactions with each patient. If that appeals to you, great, but if it doesn't then you will want to find a dentist who takes the time you need. You want your questions answered and you want to feel like you are the most important thing for him to focus on when you are in the chair. If the dentist is being pulled in many different directions, you may feel that the distractions are a bit too much and that you are not the center of attention at a time when you should be.

Getting Personal Recommendations

When you begin looking for dentist recommendations from people you know, you want to narrow down if there is a specific type of dentist you are looking for. While most people have experience with a general dentist, for example, they may not have experience with someone who specializes in cosmetic dentistry or pediatric dentistry. If you have a desire or need for a specific type of dentist, then you need to let people know that from the start, so you are not given recommendations to numerous general dentists who do not handle such areas.

It's difficult for people to recommend a specialist dentist if they haven't had experience with the person themselves. When seeking personal recommendations from people, you want to hear the direct experience that they have had with the dentist. You are trusting your smile to the dentist you choose, so you want to make sure that you are choosing the right one for your family. Ending up with someone who isn't a good fit will leave you with regrets and possibly not liking your smile. It can also leave your kids growing up with a fear of the dentist that will stick with them for a lifetime.

The dentist that your friends and family recommend may be fine for them, or they may not know much about the person either. Your friends likely don't realize the long term consequences of not having a dentist that you can trust and who will guide you in providing the best care for your family's teeth. Remember, there's more at stake here than cosmetics.

Most general dentists will offer cosmetic dentistry, and many of them do see children. But that doesn't mean they specialize on those areas, so if they are of concern to you, be sure that the dentist you choose does specialize in them. Many general dentists will not begin seeing children until they are of a certain age, usually around five or seven or so, but pediatric dentists will begin seeing children at only a year old. And if you are in need of cosmetic dentistry, you will want to choose someone who is well experienced with it, so that you get a great return on your investment.

To get recommendations from family, friends and co-workers, you could post about it on your social media networks, such as Facebook. Let people know the type of dentist you are looking for and give them an idea of location, since those who follow you are likely to cover a large geographic area. An ideal type of post if you are looking for a family dentist would be something like this:

Hello friends! Do you have a dentist you love who you would recommend? I'm looking for a new dentist for our family. We want someone who is located in our area. We need someone who will listen to us, understand our needs, and will take the time to deliver great care. Comment with your recommendation and what you love about that dentist. Thank you!

With a post like that, you are bound to get some recommendations from your friends and family. From there, you can take it further to ask questions that may come to mind, based off what they said or questions that you may have on your own. Some additional questions to consider for those giving you recommendations include:

- How long have you been going to that dentist and do your family members also love going there?
- Is there any type of specific treatments that the dentist specializes in?
- How experienced is this dentist and how much experience did you personally have with the person?
- When you need treatment, did the dentist explain what options were available to you, along with all of the advantages and disadvantages?

- When you had treatment done, how well did the dentist explain to you the procedure, so you knew what to expect? They did explain to you how long the treatment process would take and how long things like crowns would last?
- What is the dentist's policy when it comes to guarantees or protecting you if you are not happy with the treatment or if it doesn't hold up as it should?

There is a chance that the person giving you the recommendation doesn't know the answer to all of these questions. Plus, you don't necessarily want to ask them every question and grill them over the recommendations. Pick and choose which follow-up questions make sense for the recommendations you are getting, based off what they said they liked about the dentist and what you feel is appropriate to ask.

If your insurance provider gave you a list of dentists who are in their network, that may give you a referral, but it's not a quality one. They are only telling you what dentists fit their provider list, but it doesn't speak at all about what they specialize in, what their hours are like, how their personality is, and if they will be a good fit for your family.

While it's nice to have a dentist who is part of the preferred network, that approach may not always get you the best dentist for your family. Use the information as a starting point, but if you feel the best dentist for your family is not on the network list, speak to your insurance company to see what arrangements can be made. Costs and insurance plays one part of the overall picture and shouldn't be the determining factor in choosing a dentist if you want the best one for your family. Don't let fears about network lists keep you from seeking out the best dentist for your family.

Being Nice

It's important to note that you don't want to choose a dentist based on the idea that someone is nice. I once had a patient tell me that they went to a dentist's office where the hygienist was super nice. The woman was soft-spoken, friendly, and super gentle. Almost too nice if that's even possible. But the problem, as she explained it, was that when she left their office she didn't feel like her teeth were even cleaned. The woman was so mild-mannered and gentle that the patient didn't feel that her teeth got the usual cleaning that she had grown accustomed to when visiting a dentist office for a cleaning. And to make matters worse, because the woman was "nice," she didn't have the heart to say anything about it.

That's not a good situation to get into. Not only will you not be happy with the dental experience you are receiving, but you will either grow frustrated as time goes on or you will simply fade away and find a new dentist office to try. Being "nice" is great and it is necessary when working with patients, but that should not be the only criteria for which you choose a dentist office. You want nice, but you also want them to know what they are doing, be well experienced, be attentive to your wishes, and make you feel like your time there was well spent. Being nice also doesn't ensure that they specialize in the treatment options you are looking for, so look for nice, but also look beyond it to get the whole package.

Here's what I hear from many parents:

"My mom was great, but..."

"My parents were great, but..."

"...but I wish she would have gotten us a better dentist. Growing up, I was embarrassed of my mouth and would try to not show my smile. I would also cover up my mouth whenever I laughed. I didn't dare want people to see my teeth. Here I am today trying to spend a fortune to fix the problems that resulted from not getting it right to begin with."

We owe it to our family to help them get the best start that they can get. That goes for their teeth, too, since they are such an important part of someone's confidence and play such an important role in their long term health.

Advertising and Internet Referrals

Many dentists engage in advertising their services. There is nothing wrong with using advertising as a starting point in narrowing down your search for a great dentist. It should be a starting point, though, because the ad will not answer all of your questions or let you know if their personality is a good fit for your family.

One thing that advertising should do is answer a few of the questions you have regarding any specialty areas that they focus on. Most dentists who advertise will want to let readers know that they do cosmetic dentistry, sedation dentistry, pediatrics, or that they offer weekend appointments. They will want to get those key points into their ad, so they can help you narrow down your search.

If you see an advertisement for a dentist that catches your eye and gets your attention, take the info and do your additional research. You will still want to see if others you know have ever gone to the person and what their experience was like and you will want to be sure to interview the dentist and ask questions.

Today, it's common for people to begin their search for a new dentist online. While there is a ton of information regarding dentists online, there's one word to sum up how you should approach it:

Caution.
The Internet can be both great and horrible for finding a new dentist. You have immediate access to a plethora of information on the one hand, but on the other, you have no idea how valid any of it is. In today's world, there are people who pay for good reviews to be posted, you can have negative reviews posted by someone who is actually your competition, and you may have people leaving reviews on sites who have never even been near the dentist's office they are leaving a review for. In other words, take what you find online with a grain of salt and still do your in-person evaluation.

As with anything you read online, you have to consider the source. If you are at the dentist's website, you can take what is on there at face value. They are likely to provide you with truthful information about what treatments they provide, the types of payment they accept, and detailed information about the people who will be taking care of you and your family there. If you are not on the dentist's website, pay close attention to the source as to whether or not it's a well-respected site or one that anyone can post anything on a whim.

Always consider the source.

In today's high-tech world, there are many review and ranking sites online. People can go there and put in their two cents on everything from their experience at hiring a plumber to staying at a particular hotel. They seem like they could be a great thing, and often times they are if you are looking for a new restaurant to try. That's because trying out a new restaurant isn't a big investment and won't be all that costly. Even if it was a horrible meal you are not out that much, so the loss isn't so great. But take the advice on something as important as a dentist and not be happy with the choice and it could have a much bigger implication for you and your family.

If you plan to use review and ranking sites, again you should take it with a grain of salt. I know wonderful dentists with zero online reviews because they have small practices and do very little advertising. I also know average and below-average dentists who have paid online marketing services for wonderful (fake) reviews. Start your online search with the understanding that the information may not be all that accurate. Use it as a starting point, but carry on with the rest of your research just the same.

While we wait to see how the case plays out in the courtroom, there was a 3-year old child who died while having a routine dental procedure in 2017 in California. The child went in to have two teeth pulled and two others capped, but within about 30 minutes of beginning the procedure she died. And this dentist had great online reviews. This is a story that plays out somewhere in the country nearly every year, and sometimes multiple times per year. Choosing the right dentist can be a life or death matter.

Featured Dentists

Chances are you have seen dentists featured in your area either in the news or in articles in newspapers and magazines. This is a great way to be introduced to a dentist, but again, treat it as a starting point. I know many dental professionals who have been featured in articles and news stories and they often have impeccable resumes and a great fan base. But that doesn't mean that every dentist you see on the news is going to be the right one for you.

Some dentists make their way into the media coverage because the reporter has selected them due to their reputation in the local field. Some dentists may be featured because they are an advertiser on the news station or in the publication, so when they need a dental source they are called upon. Still others may be working with a public relations agency that helped them get that media spot. When a dentist works with a public relations firm, they pay them a fee so that in turn they get media exposure. This is not to say anything bad about public relations work, because it's a great thing and can help dentists get their name into the public. Yet it is good for you to understand the different ways in which some dentists may get media exposure.

Having confidence in choosing the dentist who is right for you and your family starts with having a few candidates to consider. Those candidates who make your short list may come from a variety of places, including personal recommendations from family and friends, or they may come from names you have seen in advertisements or the general media. No matter how you obtain those names that make your short list, keep in mind that they are a starting point. You still have some work to do once you have those names, but I promise you that if you stick with it and see this through, you will be happy with the choice you make.

Confidently choosing the best dentist for your family starts with putting together a short list of candidates that you will further research and evaluate in order to narrow it down to the candidate you select. Simply put, choosing the right dentist for you and your family is too big of an investment to take it lightly. Scouting out the best dentist who is a good fit for your family will help ensure happy smiles, beautiful teeth, comfortable patients, and the end to battles, tears, and fear over dentist appointments.

CHAPTER 3
Relax, We've Got Your Covered

By now you are probably feeling a bit overwhelmed at all that can happen if you don't happen to find the right dentist for your family. That's understandable, considering all that is at stake, but have no fear. You can relax, because we really do have you covered. The information you are getting in this book is invaluable to helping you be able to not only understand the importance of selecting the best dentist for your family, but in determining how to do it.

We are able to give you this information because we know. We've been there. We've done the research, we have talked to many patients over the years, and we have seen what happens when you do find the right dentist, as well as when you don't. Our careers have become our passion and we have taken the liberty to study it, learning everything we can about the need for excellent dental care.

Excellent dental care, by the way, is not something that everyone can deliver. This is true even if the person is a dentist and has had the proper schooling to be in the profession. There are certain things you can learn in the classroom, but there are things that a classroom can also never teach you. Those are often the things that set great dentists apart from those who are mediocre at best. Those characteristics are the ones that you want in the dentist that you choose for your family.

Excellent dentists have some characteristics in common that lend to their great abilities and service. Some of the characteristics of excellent dentists you want to look for include:

- How friendly is the dentist? Is the person caring and attentive to your needs and concerns? Do they take the time to answer your questions thoroughly, so you feel comfortable with the information you have received? Does the person explain the procedures so you know what to expect and what the likely outcome will be?
- Does the dentist have the training and experience that you want and need in order to have the treatments done that you desire? How long have they been in practice and what type of experience do they have? Is there anything they specialize in, such as cosmetic dentistry or pediatric dentistry?

- How will the dentist handle an emergency situation? What if the emergency happens on the weekend? Will they still see you?
- Does the dentist keep up with the latest technology and techniques? This is important if you are looking for advanced cosmetic dentistry or to help reduce discomfort during treatment.
- How much of a part of your community is the dentist? Do they give back, get involved, and seem to be a part of the community?
- How do they treat new patients in terms of being able to get appointments? Will you be waiting months to have your first appointment?
- What types of things is the dentist able to do in order to help you or someone in your family with anxiety about going to their office?

A great dentist is going to go above and beyond for every patient. Just providing you with the treatment you expected when you walked in the door is not enough. Of course that's what they should provide, but that is not going to excite you and get you loving that dentist office.

When it comes down to it, you want a dentist office that is going to remember your birthday, be involved in the community, and remember who you are by name. When you sit down in their chair, you want them to remember that you are passionate about the Dodgers, or whatever your thing is, and you want them to ask you about it. You want them to surprise you with thank you notes and for them to show gratitude that out of all the dentist offices in the area, you chose their office.

If your dentist doesn't do all of that, and most of them don't, then you are not with the right dentist. The right dentist will make you feel appreciated and that you are their only patient that day. They will give you the time you deserve, so that you understand everything, all of your questions are answered, and that you feel confident and comfortable with everything that takes place.

Everyone deserves a dentist who is going to provide them with well above average care. Anyone can provide you with average care, but you should want more than that and seek out more than that. Remember the days when you used to pull up to a gas pump and someone came to your window to see what type of service you wanted? They would wash your windows, check the air in your tire, pump your gas, and more. It was full service. Today, it's pretty much unheard of for someone to get full service like that not only in the gas industry, but pretty much anywhere.

Now imagine what it would be like for you to get "full service" so to speak at the dentist office. From the moment you step into the door you feel special, the people working there are attentive to your needs. They show appreciation for you being there, they make you feel comfortable. The waiting room is decked out in comfortable furniture, as well as some drinks for your wait. When you get called back to the room, the dentist is happy to see you, and speaks to you as if you are old friends. When your birthday rolls around you get a hand-written birthday greeting in the mail. What would such full service at the dentist office feel like? It would feel amazing, and believe me, it's out there.

Full service is what we offer, because we have you covered.

Bedside Manner Above All

Years ago, people felt that they had a better connection with their dentists and other doctors. Bedside manner, as it was referred to, was something that was at the top of the priority list for every person looking for a new dentist. Bedside manner in a nutshell is the approach that the dentist, or any other doctor, takes in their attitude toward the patient.

Bedside manner has largely become an issue most people don't speak about today, but it's something that everyone feels. Every patient feels the attitude that the dentist has toward them, whether it is one of indifference or one of gratitude. They can be caring or they can be callous and not engaged. Whether you call it bedside manner or dental chair side manner, it's still important today.

Find a dentist who has a great bedside manner and you will find that you get much more out of the relationship. You will feel like you have a connection to the dentist, and that connection is important to feeling comfortable, confident, and knowing you have the right dentist for you and your family.

Not having the right dentist for your family can be a scary thing. It can make people want to avoid the dentist and they may not get the best care even if they do go for appointments. Choosing the best dentist for your family is going to make a world of difference in your smiles, but as well as with your emotional well being. Your teeth are an investment in you, now and well into the future.

CHAPTER 4
Why is Your Smile So Important?

Have you ever thought about what you may be missing out on if you don't like your smile? What about those people who dislike their smile so much that they hide it when they laugh, or they refuse to show their teeth when they smile? What is that doing to their mental health? You may be surprised at just how much a smile is linked to when it comes to our emotional well-being and our quality of life overall.

There is plenty of research and information about how having low self esteem can cost you when it comes to jobs. Those who don't like the way they look usually have lower self esteem, and when that happens they will go to job interviews giving off those vibes.

Having low self esteem tends to make people seem that they lack the confidence to get the job done. Those who don't feel confident tend to let it show through their body language, which is something that people immediately pick up on. Not liking your smile can also have a negative impact on your job and career because you are less likely to speak up, get involved, close the deal, and take the necessary career risks that can lead you to the next level.

Those with low self esteem on the job will also lack the confidence to ask for a raise or negotiate a higher salary right from the start. As you can see, not loving your teeth is costing you. And it's costing you a lot.

Those who fear the costs of investing in their smile should consider the high cost of not investing in their smile.

Self image is extremely important in most areas of our life. How we feel about ourselves has an impact on our interpersonal relationships, schoolwork, peer relationships, careers, and more. Something as small as a great smile can have a major impact on many areas of your life.

It is imperative that you choose the right dentist for your family. Too much is at stake not to.

Liking your smile is not something beyond your reach. It's well within your reach for you and your family, and it's something that everyone deserves. When you like your teeth and smile, you are going to have a much better time in life, be happier, and will be putting your best foot forward when it comes to helping your child get better grades and helping them get a good start in the adult future. You will be helping yourself to improve your quality of life, further your career, and make better connections with those around you.

The Science Behind a Smile

Now that you know the impact that a great smile has on everything, let's dig a little deeper. There is a lot of science behind how important a great smile is in one's life, too. There's a lot that goes on behind the scenes when it comes to smiles, and it's something that most people never even consider.

Have you ever noticed that when you smile at people they tend to smile back? Smiles can be contagious. People smile, which leads to more people smiling, which leads to a happier community and nicer place to live. There is a lot of research out there about the importance of a smile, such as when we meet strangers. Our brains are essentially hard-wired to not have favorable opinions when we first lay our eyes on strangers. This is a primitive defense mechanism that works to help keep us safe. But the interesting thing here is that a smile immediately changes that signal in the brain. When you see the smile on a person's face, it immediately sends a signal to the brain that turns the signal from foe to friend.

That's how powerful a smile is.

Smiling affects your brain, your attitude, and the way people respond to you. It's part of body language, and you have probably heard before how important body language is to communication overall. We do most of our communicating with our body language. It's amazing how well woven into our life a smile really is and the impact that it has on us and those around us.

Internally, there is something incredible that happens with a simple smile. When you smile, it helps to relieve stress, because your brain releases what are called neuropeptides. The transmitters that are released are endorphins, serotonin, and dopamine, all of which make us feel good. One quick smile on your face, and your brain immediately goes into action releasing these feel-good chemicals into your body that make you happy.

Did you know that you don't have to actually be happy for the smile to have this impact? You can force the smile and have it lead to happiness, rather than the other way around. The next time you feel down, force yourself to hold a smile on your face for about two minutes. Sure, it's a fake smile that you are forcing, but here's the thing: Your brain doesn't realize that. Your brain gets the signal that there is a smile on your face and ding, ding, ding, it starts pumping out the feel-good chemicals. Next thing you know your mood is lifted, you feel better, and your stress level has diminished.

In other words, when it comes to smiling, you can fake it until you make it.

The endorphins that are released by your brain when you are smiling act as a natural pain reliever in your body. The serotonin works to lift your mood so that you don't feel sad or depressed, serving as a natural built-in antidepressant. Consider how many people take prescription pain pills and antidepressants every year. Smiling more can help keep pain and depression away, as well as help people avoid these costly drugs that have potentially harmful side effects.

Since smiling releases these important feel-good chemicals in the body, it can help to transform your life and that of those around you. When you feel happier, you are going to be in a better mood with those around you, helping to improve their quality of life and add to their happiness. So much is tied to the smile, yet so many people let time go by without putting one on their face.

Smiling is what is considered an active expression. It's one that draws people in and engages others. Think about it: When is the last time you saw someone with a pinch-faced look or an angry face and it made you want to engage with that person? Most likely not often, because if you see someone like that your initial reaction is going to be to head the other direction or avoid engaging them. But if you see someone smiling, that active expression is more inviting and there is a good chance you will engage. You will either smile back, say a few words, or just make friendly eye contact.

People are drawn toward those who have friendly faces and who are smiling. The more you like your smile and your teeth, the more likely you are to have a smile on your face more often. This is going to make you feel more comfortable interacting with others. Smiling helps you connect with others in a happy and positive manner, and that's something we can all use. Showing a beautiful smile and teeth makes you look friendlier, more relaxed, happier, and more approachable to those around you. This goes for you, as well as your children, who are at a vulnerable period for making friends and connecting with others.

There's Even More Science

Researchers tend to do studies on a broad range of topics each year, but it's no surprise that they have done so much on the act of smiling. Even before we had the scientific proof to back it up, we all kind of knew the importance of a smile and how it can impact your life. We have all felt it, we see it, and it's something that is universal. Even if you don't understand someone else's language, a smile is something we can all understand. We know that it's a friendly gesture that is meant to show a good nature.

When endorphins are released when we smile it makes us feel happier, but it also helps to relieve stress. We know that stress in our body can lead to some major health issues, such as cardiovascular disease. The cortisol in our body is active when we feel stressed or anxious, but it's combated when the endorphins are released from smiling.

Smiling is actually good for your overall health, too.

We also know that laughing is good for us, even improving the body's homeostasis. The first step to laughing is a good old fashioned smile. You can't laugh without smiling. They go hand-in-hand. Laughing brings oxygen into the body, releases stress and tension, and helps keep us healthy. Laughing also helps us to release emotions, so if you have something on your mind that is causing distress, you can have a good laugh and that will all ease away.

Smiling not only lifts your mood and helps you to be a happier person, but it helps to improve your immune system. A smile literally creates chemical changes within the body that strengthen your immune system, thus helping to keep you from getting sick and being able to fight off viruses quicker. Doctors have even seen the power of a smile when they take someone's blood pressure. Smiling before getting blood pressure taken helps to lower the rate and give you a better reading.
Finally, it's important to state one of the obvious reasons that a smile is so important, and that's because it makes us more attractive. People tend to look younger, friendlier, and more attractive when they smile.

But there is one caveat here, which is that having great teeth kicks it up a notch. Those who smile and have obvious teeth problems won't shine as being as attractive as they would if they had great teeth.

Beautiful people all have one thing in common: a beautiful smile.

Although there is a lot of science and research that tells us about the inner workings and mechanics of a smile, all of these things solidify what we already feel. They let us know that yes, a smile is a major component to living a happy life and that it does great things for us both internally and externally. But we already know intrinsically how important a smile is. This is because it's something we live. When you look in the mirror and smile or you see someone else smiling, you already know the importance that has in your life. You don't need a scientist to tell you that it's good for you, because you can feel that it's good for you. It's nice to have research back up what we know, but in all honesty it's not telling us anything that we don't already feel and see for ourselves.

Dale Carnegie, writer of the famous book called "How to Win Friends and Influence People," also knew about the importance of a smile. He knew that smiling is an important part to both winning friends and being able to have the power to influence people. One of the things he said about the importance of a smile was:

"A smile costs nothing, but creates much. It enriches those who receive, without impoverishing those who give. It happens in a flash and the memory of it sometimes lasts forever."

Dean Martin hit the nail on the head when he said that when you smile, the whole world smiles with you. That's one of the best ways to look at it. Do you want the world smiling with you? Then you need to smile more, and to smile more you have to love your smile. One of the most effective ways for you and your family members to love their smile is to make sure you choose the right dentist for your family.

Peace of Mind

One of the most important reasons for helping to ensure your family members have a smile that they like is, well, peace of mind. Without a doubt, you want the best for everyone in your family, or you wouldn't be reading this book to begin with. No parent wants their child to suffer, especially from teeth that hurt, embarrass them, or cause social problems. But the fact is that their formative years are some of the most important ones for their development now and into adulthood.

Ensuring that you choose the right dentist helps you to give your family the very best foundation for a great smile. As you know, a smile is so important to our development, our success, and in our quality of life. The number one thing we all want in life is happiness, and you cannot have that without a smile.

Giving your kids, and yourself, a great smile by having the best possible dentist for your family, is a gift. It's a gift that will help them in many ways, physically and emotionally. It's also one that brings peace of mind, and that's something we can all appreciate.

A great smile is the foundation of a happy life. A great smile brings peace of mind.

CHAPTER 5
Is a Great Smile Just a Cosmetic Issue?

In order to be successful in life, you need to feel good about the way you look, and liking your smile is a huge part of that. Not having a great smile can lead to everything from missed job opportunities and lower salaries to not cultivating great interpersonal relationships. When you think about all the damage that can be done to someone's emotional well-being simply because they don't like their smile or teeth, it's clear to see how important the topic is. Your family's smiles and teeth are simply something that cannot be ignored.

But is a great smile just a cosmetic issue? Is there more to the story than what meets the eye with every smile? You better believe there is. There's a lot more at stake here than just the cosmetic issue. The cosmetic issue alone is a major area of concern, as I've been sharing in the previous chapters. There is no mistaking how essential it is that people like their teeth and their smile. Going beyond cosmetics, there are plenty of other reasons to make sure that your teeth and smile, and that of those in your family, is great.

Your health also depends on having a great smile and well cared-for teeth, making it crucial that you put a lot of thought into choosing the right dentist. It's too important of an issue to simply throw a dart at the wall and hope that the little tip ends up on a great option. That may occasionally work for some people, but for the majority it is not going to be a good route to take. Not everyone is great at throwing darts, and when you haven't been the one to set up the options on the board, you don't know if hitting any particular candidate's picture is going to be better than another's.

Misaligned, "Crooked" Teeth Equal Significant Medical Problems.
Poorly aligned teeth can produce chronic headaches and migraines, contribute to digestive problems because of poor chewing of foods, make getting a decent night's sleep impossible, and, maybe most dangerous, foster gum disease. Gum disease has absolute links to diabetes, heart disease, strokes and dementia, as well as, of course, loss of natural teeth altogether. Orthodontic corrections later in adult life are more difficult, can be painful, require time off work, and at best, can themselves be an embarrassment.

Uncorrected mouth problems and misaligned teeth make for strangely stretched gums inevitably destined to separate from teeth and allow "pockets" for infections and periodontal disease that turns into VERY difficult and painful and costly problems late in life.

Gum disease is serious business. It worsens risks of and heightens dangers from diabetes, heart disease, strokes and dementia.

Perhaps you are thinking that nobody in your family has any significant dental issues. Okay, while I can't say for sure because I haven't done an examination to see if there are underlying issues that need to be corrected, for the sake of this discussion we will go with it. Well, tooth alignment treatment aside, there are still many reasons why having a great dentist is crucial to your overall health. Let's start by talking about periodontal disease.

Nasty Periodontal Disease

If you haven't heard it before, let me be the first to tell you that periodontal disease is nasty. And you and your family members do not want it. In fact, you want to stay as far away from it as possible. If you don't already know what it is, then the more you learn about it the more likely are to agree that it's something you want to steer clear of now and long into the future.

Periodontal disease is typically what results from inflammation and infections that take place in the gums and the bones that surround the teeth. In the early stages of periodontal disease, it starts out as gingivitis. During this state, the gums become inflamed and red, as well as swollen. You may also find that they bleed when you brush your teeth. Left untreated, gingivitis will continue to advance, wreaking havoc on your mouth.

When you have gingivitis that is allowed to advance, it can end up making your gums pull away from the teeth. That is simply nothing to mess with. What do you think happens when the gums pull away from the teeth? Well, the gums are a big part of what is holding the teeth in your mouth, so when they pull away you risk losing teeth.

With gingivitis, you begin to see the destruction just getting started. The redness, inflammation, and some bleeding gums is a huge sign there is a problem that needs to be addressed immediately. It's going to get worse if it doesn't get treated. But left untreated, as it continues to advance it moves into a stage called periodontitis. It's in this stage that the gums pull away from the teeth. This causes the teeth to loosen and possibly fall out.

One of the biggest threats to your oral health is periodontal disease.

Without consistent dental care, gum disease can easily creep in when you least expect it. Here's something that will knock your socks off – according to the Centers for Disease Control and Prevention, just over 47% of all adults who are over the age of 30 have some form of periodontal disease.

Thank about that for a moment. Nearly half of all adults in the country are walking around with a disease that can lead to their gums bleeding and pulling away from their teeth, and their teeth loosening and falling out of their mouth. This is serious stuff. And it doesn't get better; the stats actually get worse as you age. By the time adults reach the age of 65, 70% of them have periodontal disease.

Here are a few more statistics from the American College of Prosthodontists that show you just how important of an issue taking care of your teeth is:

- More than 36 million Americans don't have any teeth. Let that sink in for a minute. There are 36 million people in this country who don't have any teeth at all.
- Tooth loss happens from decay and gum disease, which can be a result of wear, cancer, injury, etc.
- Of those who have no teeth, around 90% of them have dentures.
- They estimate that the problem of toothlessness will continue to grow to more than 200 million people within the next 15 years.

It may seem as though it's a simple issue. When you lose teeth, you just go get dentures. But it's not that simple. Not at all and actually far from it. There are some serious health problems that can arise from having missing teeth, which many people find surprising.

Some of the consequences of missing teeth can include nutritional changes, some forms of cancer, coronary artery disease, and obesity. These are serious problems that can arise from missing teeth, so it's imperative to try to take the best possible care of your teeth throughout your life, and that includes by finding the right dentist for you and your family and then visiting regularly for check-ups and any necessary treatments that are recommended to you.

In a 2013 study that was published in the International Journal of Dentistry, researchers explained the connection between oral health and a person's overall general health. In their report, they stated that despite there being advances in preventative dentistry, people losing their teeth (called edentulism) was still a major worldwide health problem.

Some of the key findings from their important study include:

· Edentulism is both debilitating and irreversible. Once someone loses their adult teeth, they cannot reverse that and go back.
· They report that edentulism is more popular among women.
· Studies show that denture wearing continues to increase.

When it comes to how tooth loss impacts overall general health, the researchers report that tooth loss was also associated with eating an unhealthy diet, it increased rates of chronic inflammatory changes of the gastric mucosa, and led to higher rates of peptic ulcers. Those who are missing their teeth also have higher rates of diabetes mellitus, hypertension, heart failure, stroke, sleep apnea, and chronic kidney disease. Furthermore, tooth loss was also associated with a decrease in being physically active and leading a healthy quality of life.

That's an incredible amount of problems that can arise from not taking the best possible care of your teeth. Sure, some of these problems may happen anyway, even if you do try to take good care of your teeth, but by having the best possible dentist, going for regular appointments, and getting treatments as they are needed, you will be doing a great deal to help lower those risks.

Does all of this scare the living hell out of you? Well, in all honesty it's something that should do exactly that. Far too often, we go through life not discussing the implications of some of the decisions we make. There are millions of people who don't realize how important their teeth are and the best possible way to care for them until it's too late. Don't be one of those people. Armed with the knowledge of why having the best oral care impacts your health, even beyond just cosmetic reasons, it's important to take that information and put it into action. Stop at nothing short of your family having the best possible dentist, who will help you reduce the risks of problems, recommend treatments that are necessary, and will help you continue to have a higher quality of life.

Our teeth play a major role in our lives. They may be small, but their impact is tremendous. Taking care of them and finding the best dentist for us and our family is paramount.

Tooth Decay

There's another dirty little area that we need to talk about when it comes to tooth care beyond the cosmetics. That's the area of tooth decay.

There's no doubt that you are likely familiar with what cavities are. They are holes in the teeth. But did you know that cavities start from tooth decay? A cavity isn't something that happens overnight. Rather, it is a process that takes place little by little over time.

The good news here is that tooth decay can be stopped, as well as reversed. This will help keep you and your family from getting cavities. But if regular dental visits are not being kept up, then tooth decay is allowed to continue getting worse until one day your child has a tooth that keeps hurting, you take them to a dentist and find out that they have a cavity. Next, you are crossing your fingers that the cavity was found in a state small enough that you can get away with just filling it, rather than needing something more, such as a root canal or crown.

The longer tooth decay is left unaddressed, the more damage it does. The longer cavities are left untreated the more damage they do, and the more it will cost you to repair it. Plus, you can't reverse a cavity. Once the hole is there, it's there forever and you can only do something to fill or cover it. Tooth decay caught early can be addressed and the teeth can be better protected from reaching the state of having a cavity.

It's estimated that 25% of the adult population in the country has untreated tooth decay.

Consider that for a moment, one out of every four adults who are reading this book is doing so with untreated tooth decay. You may not even be aware that you have it, but it's there, lurking in your mouth, just waiting to wreak havoc on your teeth. Unless you take action to find the best dentist and start getting treatment for that tooth decay, your future will have cavities in it, as well as possibly have crowns, root canals, and possibly even tooth loss.

Our mouths are filled with bacteria, and some of it can be harmful to the teeth. If you drink a lot of drinks with sugar in them, or if you eat a lot of starchy foods (cookies, crackers, chips), those create a plaque on the teeth that will lead to mineral loss and tooth decay. The bacteria in your mouth use the sugar and starches to produce acid that eats away at the teeth, starting the downward spiral.

When teeth are repeatedly exposed to the acid attacks, the enamel will continue to lose minerals. Over time, more minerals are lost, and the enamel becomes weak and a hole is created, which is the cavity. Don't let this happen to you and your family, because it can be prevented and reversed.

When the acid that is produced attacks your teeth, it's bad news. That's where you will begin to have tooth decay that can lead to something even worse. That is unless you are seeing a great dentist so that they can help you address it, and reverse the process. Tooth decay can absolutely be treated, but time is of the essence. Getting it addressed immediately is the only way to help ensure that it doesn't spread deeper into the teeth. Left untreated or ignored, the damage will continue to mount.

Makes a Great Window

Many health professionals believe that your oral health is literally a window to your overall health. People who have poor oral health are at a higher risk for having poor health in other areas. We've discussed some of them, but here's a quick rundown of some of the issues that poor oral health is believed to contribute to:

- Cardiovascular disease – oral inflammation is believed to increase risks of heart attack and stroke.
- Premature birth and low birth weight – it's estimated that around 18% of preterm births and low birth weight babies are attributed to mothers having oral infections.
- Poorly controlled diabetes – poor oral health may make it more difficult to control diabetes.

Periodontitis is believed to be linked to numerous health problems and diseases. Plus, poor oral health can lead to a lower quality of life, both mentally and physically. The saliva in your mouth is like a fingerprint. It's that important and can be useful in gathering information about your overall health, as well as for drug testing, hormonal changes, and to test for various diseases. Our mouths and oral health can reveal so much about us, it really does make a great window to our overall health.

Research has been conducted that has shown that bacteria that that is associated with gum disease can increase inflammation and raise cholesterol levels. The bacteria can also travel from the mouth to the liver, lungs, kidneys, and heart. This is something that we don't think much about, but it can have a huge impact on our lives and our overall health.

Many people who already have health problems may also be more prone to oral health issues. Certain prescriptions can negatively impact oral health by reducing the amount of saliva that is produced. Some of the disease that can contribute to oral health problems include diabetes, HIV/AIDS, osteoporosis, eating disorders, rheumatoid arthritis, neck and head cancers, and Alzheimer's disease.

Anyone trying to maintain good overall health should never overlook oral health. The links between the two are profound and the research has shown the many connections. It's important to make sure that you and your family receive the best possible dental care so that you can help to lower the risks of getting a wide variety of diseases over time.

Oral health is often overlooked by people who are on a quest to be healthy. They tend to start exercising and go on a diet, but they remain unaware of the strong connection between their oral health and their general health overall. Armed with this information, you can use it to help keep you and your family much healthier.

Not Merely Cosmetic

As you can see after reading this chapter, a great smile is not just a cosmetic issue. Not by a long shot. In fact, it would be difficult to say which is more important, the psychological health that comes from a great smile, or the overall general health that comes from it. You need both in order to live a well-balanced life that is considered high quality. If you have one without the other you, will be missing out on a lot in your life.

Having a great smile is so much more than just loving what you see in the mirror or in pictures. It's also about the things we can't see with the naked eye, such as what the bacteria in our mouths are doing and how they are impacting the rest of our body. Take care of your oral health and you will be doing a lot of good in helping to take care of your overall health.

With your oral health being such a significant contributor to your overall health and quality of life, it's imperative that you find the right dentist for your family. The right dentist will be an ally, armed with the tools and knowledge you need on your side, to help keep you and your family healthier.

CHAPTER 6
Why Not Just Any Dentist?

What a wonderful world it would be if we could all just trust the fact that any dentist we called up to make an appointment with was a great one. That would be fantastic, because then we wouldn't have to worry about anything happening that we hadn't bargained for when we made the decision to sit down in their chair. Unfortunately, that's not the world that we live in, and it's likely never going to be.

Believe it or not, there are dentists who lose their license, have many complaints filed against them, and who make the news for their horrible practices.

The last thing you want is to have made an appointment with a dentist that you regret. As an adult, you may be a little more understanding in that if you go to a dentist who isn't a good fit, you can move on to find another one. But kids are not so easily forgiving in this regard. If you take your child to a dentist who is a lousy fit, you could be setting them up to never want to go to a dentist again. They may immediately form the opinion that it's scary, painful, and something to be avoided at all costs.

Right now, you are helping to lay the foundation for how your children will go through their life addressing their oral care. Several years back, I had a conversation with a man who was around 40 years old and needed something done to one of his teeth because he was in pain. He was the type of person who had been largely avoiding the dentist his entire adult life, only finally breaking down to go in when there was something bothering him to the point that he couldn't take it anymore.

We discussed why it is that he doesn't go to the dentist regularly. He was an intelligent man who understands the importance of good oral care. He realizes that it's important to go to the dentist regularly, so it didn't make a lot of sense why he wasn't going. And this was the example he was setting for his children, who see how often Dad goes to the dentist (or doesn't in this case). So I dug a little deeper to inquire as to why he isn't going regularly, despite him knowing the importance of it. Then he explained and it all made a whole lot of sense.

When this man was a child, he grew up poor and on welfare. His parents took him to the health department of a major city for the dental work that he needed. He wasn't taken there regularly or for teeth cleanings, but typically only when there was a problem. When he was a teenager he recalls the how the dentist made him feel so bad, because he sat there saying things to him like "I can't believe what a mess your teeth are, you have so many problems." The dentist went on and on saying things to him like this, essentially shaming him, yet he was in the office seeking help.

The shame and humiliation this man felt as a young teen laid the groundwork for the relationship he has with dentists today. First of all, he's ashamed to go to the dentist. He feels as though instead of the dentist helping him by providing treatment and being on his side, that he is judging him and is disgusted with his teeth. Secondly, when he was growing up he was only taken to the dentist when there was a problem, so he continues that path today. He was taught that when you have pain or a problem that won't go away, that's when you finally break down and go to the dentist.

This man doesn't know what it's like to go in for a routine check-up or cleaning. He has been conditioned to think that the dentist is going to humiliate him because he doesn't have great teeth, and that he only needs to go to him as a last resort because the pain or problem won't go away. This is a sad, sad, situation that not only impacts him, but it impacts others, because there is a good chance that his children will grow up to follow in their dad's footsteps. This man's father may have even had the same relationship with dentists while he was growing up, and the cycle continues.

His poor relationship today is a result of what happened to him at the dentist office while he was growing up. While the individual problems may vary, this type of story is repeated among adults around the country. You wouldn't believe how many adults are fearful of the dentist, distrust them, or avoid them, because of the experiences that they had starting out as children.

First Impressions Matter

We all know in life how important first impressions are. We want to believe that we don't judge things on a first impression and in such a quick manner, but the truth of the matter is that our brains are hardwired to do so. Our brains are hardwired to make immediate judgment calls on something and file the information away about whether it was something good, bad, to be feared, etc. This goes back to our early ancestors, when our brains had to immediately help us to decipher mortal danger. Being able to make immediate judgment calls helped to save our lives. It told us whether we needed to act on our fight or flight instincts.

Today, we do the same thing even when we make that first visit at the dentist office. First impressions go a long way, especially when you are a child visiting the dentist for the first time. You are taking in the sights, the smells, the way the dentist speaks to you, and whether or not what they are doing scares or hurts you. Your brain is building a file, labeled "dentist," where all of this information is being quickly written and stored. What goes into that file is crucial to how you will feel about dentists going forward.

Imagine for a moment how different things would have turned out for the man I was speaking about if he had gone to a dentist who would have made a better impression on him. What if the dentist would have been more professional, had a better attitude, and looked out for the best interest of this child? Even if the child had sat in his chair and when he peered into his mouth what he saw was a cause for alarm, things could have turned out differently if the dentist had been more professional. What if he had been more gentle with him, helped him to not feel ashamed, and led him to believe that the dentist was on his side, that he was going be with him as a united front to help treat his teeth and help him get to a point where he loved his teeth?

What an incredible difference this dentist would have made in that young person's life. He would have helped lay a healthy foundation for what the person thought about dentists. He would have explained to him why it was important for him to go for regularly visits to the dentist, rather than waiting until the pain and discomfort forced him into making an appointment. And since this man would have likely had a different relationship with the dentist as an adult, he would have set a different example for his children, who also would have grown up with a better and healthier view of the dentist.

Believe me, who you choose as your dentist has a profound impact.

Knowing how important good dental care is for your oral health, as well as for your emotional one, it just makes sense that not any dentist will do. Anyone can go to school to complete the necessary coursework to become a dentist. But not just anyone can be a great dentist. Along with the dental skills and knowledge, it takes people skills to also be a great dentist. You deserve a great dentist, and so does everyone in your family.

Making sure you have the best possible dentist for your family is an act of love. It helps to ensure their oral health needs will be met, which will be a great step toward helping to provide a safeguard for their emotional and overall general health. It's a small act that has a big and effective outcome. There is simply too much at stake when it comes to oral health to just go to any dentist. It's imperative that you and your family have the best one, someone who will put your best interests in the forefront, and who understands people, as well as oral health. A great dentist is a bit like a super hero, because the job they do is that damned important.

Let's take a look at a few more reasons why not just any dentist will do. The internet has made it easy and efficient to get news from around the world. Decades ago, you only saw the news stories that made it to your local or national news, and let's be honest, it was a small fraction of what was really going on in the world. It was likely extremely rare that you ever heard the horror stories of what can happen when you don't have a great dentist. Today, that's all changed.

In today's news-filled world, it's easy to see what's going on in the dental world. You can quickly gain the latest research or read up on the best way to handle a minor discomfort. But you can also do a quick news search to see what the questionable dentists around the world are up to, because they make the headlines for those who are paying attention to them.

Do a couple of quick online searches and you are sure to find some of the dentist horror stories that have made the news in recent years. There are stories ranging from dentists being accused of harming and even torturing children, to those who did more work than they were supposed to, and some who did more harm than good. Some of the stories are enough to send shivers up your spine. I have no idea of the final outcome of the charges alleged in each of these news stories, but there's no doubt that there are some shady dentists out there.

Your mission is to find a dentist who isn't shady. You want to find a dentist who is the complete opposite and is considered excellent all the way around. Anything short of that and you will be selling you and your family short. The excellent dentists exist, trust me. It's just a matter of you opting for them to be your oral care partner. Once you do that, everything else will fall right into place.

Always remember that first impressions matter and can have a lifelong impact on how your children grow up to view dentists.

Professionalism Matters
The dentist who is right for you and your family is one who is going to be professional in all areas of providing care. They will speak to you in a caring and open manner; they will maintain professionalism throughout every appointment; they will value your time; and they will be honest. Being able to trust your dentist is important so that you know the treatment being proposed is necessary and that you feel comfortable with all of the information you have received about it.

Along with professionalism, there are other factors that you need to consider when choosing a dentist. If at least most of these other areas don't fall into place with what you are looking for in a dental office, then obviously it is not a good fit. While you may have to compromise on something, you don't want to compromise on a lot, and you don't want to compromise on the bigger and more important issues. If you do compromise on the most important issues, you will spend time regretting it and likely soon be back to the drawing board to find another dentist.

Some of the other factors that demonstrate that not just any dentist will do for you and your family include:

- **Qualifications.** This should be a given, but the dentist's qualification are going to make a big difference. In order to have a great experience, you need a competent dentist. You need one who has the education, skills, and experience to provide you and your family with great care.

- **Location.** Where the dentist is located is going to make a difference to you. Everyone has a certain amount of time they are comfortable putting in to drive back and forth to the dentist. Beyond that, they will be close to the point of losing it, because they won't want to put the time in. Choosing a dentist who is in a geographic area you are comfortable with is going to help lay the foundation for a good relationship.

- **Hours.** Once you have the office location nailed down, it will be important that they offer hours that will work for you and your family. If you know you always need evening appointments, then it's clear to see that just any dentist won't do. You will have to seek out the ones who offer the hours that will work for you and start your evaluation of those candidates there.

- **Expenses.** Most people have concerns regarding the cost of going to the dentist. Whether you have dental insurance or not, you want to make sure that the dentist you choose is going to be a good fit when it comes to costs. Make sure they accept your insurance or work with them, or if you are self-pay, find out if they accept such patients and what their terms are. Some dentists will give you a discount for being self-pay.

- **Emergency care.** Not just every dentist offers emergency care options. The last thing you want is to have a tooth knocked out, call your dentist, and get a recording or answering service that just tells you to go to the emergency room. A great dentist is going to want to be there to help you through those emergency situations.

- **Your comfort.** How comfortable you and your family members are when walking into a dentist office is important. When you walk into the right dentist's office you want to feel welcome, appreciated, and comfortable. You want to be comfortable not just with the dentist, but with the hygienist and those who work in the office. Everyone should make you feel welcome and appreciated. Anything short of that just won't do.

- **Atmosphere.** Not just any dentist will do when it comes to the office atmosphere. Each year, there are complaints lodged to professional boards regarding particular dentist offices being dirty, for example. Once these boards receive the complaints they do go out and inspect the offices, but it's one more example of how just any dentist won't do. You do not want to get oral care treatment in a place that is dirty. The dental office you go to should be impeccably clean, which helps to protect your health.

- **Complaints.** In addition to the complaints that official boards receive regarding dentist offices being filthy, they also get other complaints from the public. While some complaints may not be founded and could be bogusly filed, it's important to be aware if the dentist office has received many complaints, what they were filed for, and what the final outcome of them was. It's just one more piece of the puzzle in determining the best possible dentist for your family.

Believe it or not, there are even complaints filed each year regarding various dentist's personalities. The problem here is that while there are professional ethics that dentists should follow, there are no rules and regulations regarding one's personality. A governing board, for example, cannot tell a dentist that he or she needs a more pleasant attitude or a better personality. There's no guidelines about what your personality should be like, and it's not typically something that is taught in dental school.

The issue about the dentist's personality, however, is an important one. That's one more reason why just any dentist won't do. You need a dentist who has a personality that you are going to like. While it would be amazing to have someone who's personality is out of this world, you may not be able to find that, but you should be able to find someone who has a nice personality. You should have no problem finding someone who knows how to treat their patients well and show them that they appreciate having them as patients.

You want to know how I think patients should be treated? Well, in our offices we believe every patient should be treated like family. That's right. I want people to feel like they know us, to feel comfortable, and to feel a sense of belonging. If we set out to treat every patient like family, then we will be giving them the kind of treatment that we want to receive.

You deserve the same type of great treatment that a dentist would give his or her own family members, and nothing short of it.

In later chapters, we will go into more detail of what to look for when choosing a great dentist. Yet this gives you an idea of how important it is to not select just any dentist, because quite honestly not just any dentist will do.

Finding the right dentist is more than just opening the phone book or taking the advice of one friend. There is more that goes into it, and not everyone's situation is the same. Your family is unique, which means your situation is unique, which means you need a dentist that will be right for your unique family.

If you were to ask 10 people if they have any dental horror stories, there is a good chance that at least half of them will have something to share. Maybe it was a botched treatment, a missed issue, something they felt was done that didn't need to be done, a dentist who made them feel ashamed, or a dentist who made them afraid to see dentists regularly. The horror stories regarding dental care are vast. The best way to help prevent them from becoming stories that your family goes on to share is by doing everything within your power to find the best possible dentist for you and your family.

Vow to end the dental horror stories here and now. Make the commitment to helping your family have the best dental and oral health experience. This will help serve them now and well into the future, as well as helping to lay the foundation for future generations to also have a good dental experience.

CHAPTER 7
How to Know What Questions to Ask

Imagine getting a flyer in the mail from a new dentist office that has opened up three minutes from your home. The postcard looks nice and if offers an introductory special for new patients. It's enough to entice you to make an appointment, so you waste no time in getting it set up for the next week. Great, they got you into an appointment quickly, but does that mean you are all set and everything is going to go well?

Not so fast. A postcard that promotes a dentist may or may not be promoting the right dentist for you. And that goes for any other form of advertising or how the dentist office's information came your way to begin with. That person being advertised or referred to you by your best friend may be the best dentist in the world for you. Or maybe not. The only way you will know for sure is to dig a little deeper.

Choosing the right dentist for your family means you must ask questions and get them all answered so that you can make an informed decision.

Let's say the day of that appointment arrives that you were able to make so quickly and you go into their office. Upon walking in, you see the lobby is a bit dirty with cobwebs in the corner, outdated magazines on the tables, and a receptionist who doesn't acknowledge you. While you may be ready to withhold judgment so far, it could get worse. Maybe you go back into the exam room only to feel like you are being rushed around, without anyone caring who you are, what your name is or welcoming you as a new patient. The dentist walks in and it sends a chill up your spine because it feels like a cold front just moved in, again leaving you to wonder if you made the right decision.

The minute you start talking to the dentist about a cosmetic issue you want to get done, you have to go no further to realize you made a big mistake. The dentist gives you the vibe that they clearly are not an expert at cosmetic dentistry and don't have the experience you want or need to handle your situation. You could run out of the office, but you fear tripping on the way you, causing a scene, or simply don't want to embarrass yourself like that. So you stick it out, only to feel you wasted your time on the way home, because you feel like it's back to the drawing board with searching for the right dentist for you and your family.

Without asking questions and getting everything you need answered, there is a good chance that you will not hit a home run and find the right dentist with limited effort. It would be fantastic if you would throw a dart at some names of dentists on the wall and whichever one it lands on was the right one. It would be equally fantastic if you could find that postcard from a dentist in your mailbox, make an appointment, and when you showed up everything felt great and you knew you were in the right place.

But that's just not how it usually happens. Nope, finding the right dentist takes a little more work than that. One thing it absolutely takes is asking some questions. You can't possibly know if someone is the right dentist for you if you haven't asked some questions. And the questions that you ask are going to help make a world of difference in ensuring that you choose the right one for you and your family.

Many people cringe at the thought of going through a series of questions with the dental office they are considering. They think it's going to take up a lot of time, be obtrusive, uncomfortable, and they would rather do 100 other different things than spend their time doing that. I totally get that, but this is an area you cannot compromise on. Trust me when I say that asking the questions will actually save you a lot of time and discomfort in the long run.

Never feel bad about asking questions when you are choosing a dentist, or any doctor for that matter. This is one the most important aspects to being your best advocate. Patients must be their own best advocate, as it is the only way you will get the care that you are comfortable with and find a dentist that is a good fit for you. If you don't ask questions, you will never know if the dentist is the right one for your family.

Must-Haves for Great Dental Care
Before we even get to the set of questions you will want to ask every dental office you are considering, there are some things that I consider are "must-haves" in order for you to be getting great dental care. And you should not be settling for anything less than great dental care. Good or good enough care won't do, because there are great dentists out there who will do better than that. You deserve them, and they deserve you.

Here are the 4 must-haves that I believe must be present in order for you and your family to receive great dental care:

- **They care about you and your family.** The last thing you want is to just be another number or face that they don't remember, or where the staff is in a hurry to get you in and out of the office. You want to feel that they value and appreciate having your family there and that your treatment is important.

- **They are accessible when you need them.** It may be easy for an office to say they are going to work only Monday through Friday up until 5 p.m., but that may not be very convenient for you as a patient. What happens if your child needs a later appointment due to your job, or if there is a problem with their teeth that happens to creep up on a Saturday afternoon? Part of getting great dental treatment is that you are able to be seen and heard when you need to be. That doesn't mean the doctor should be available at your every whim, of course, but there needs to be some flexibility there. The dentist should understand the needs of busy families who may at times need an appointment in the off hours, or who have questions after hours.

- **They are forthcoming in answering your questions to give you all of the information you need.** In order for you to make decisions and feel like an active part of the treatment, you need to know and understand what is going on. A great dentist never leaves you hanging with questions or uncertainty. You should always feel comfortable with what is going on, have an understanding of why things are being done the way they are, and feel as though all of your questions are answered. The questions you have should always be welcomed and addressed. If you have a dentist who seems too busy to answer you and you feel is too brief to actually provide you with the answers you are seeking, that could be a red flag.

- **They are open and honest with you about the treatment options.** You should be able to easily obtain information about such things as cleanings, examinations, fillings, braces, and much more. Along with the information and recommendations on these things, you should also be able to easily obtain information about what the treatments will cost and the types of finance options that are available to your family.

Remember, you are investing your time into taking your family to the dentist, and there is a lot that hangs in balance. It is crucial that you get great care to ensure that your investment pays off. When you have the right dentist by your side, it should feel like a partnership. You are both working together to help ensure that your child has their dental needs met in a satisfactory manner, with both of you doing your part.

When researching a dentist for your family, it is important to make sure that you verify they are board certified. When you have one in mind whom you are considering, set up a consultation with them. When you go into the office, pay attention to how you and your children are treated. From the greeting you get at the front desk through the appointment with the doctor, you should feel welcome and comfortable.

Be sure to ask questions at that initial meeting so you know if this is the dentist you want to spend years seeing. It's also a good idea to see if there are reviews of the dentist's office online, and check with the Better Business Bureau to learn more about the reputation the office has.

What Questions to Ask

Asking questions where the dentist's office is located and if they are accepting new patients is always helpful, but your series of questions can't stop there. You need a lot more information to be able to evaluate each office you are considering. Asking the right questions will get you the answers you need to be able to evaluate, compare, and determine which dentist's office is the right one. Knowing the right questions to ask is going to help make it simple for you to narrow down the best dentist for you.

Here are some of the questions that you will want to ask every dentist's office that you interview for the position of your new family dentist:

1. **Is the dentist licensed and board certified?**
   You would think that if they are claiming to be a dentist that this is a given, that they must be licensed and possibly even be board certified. Yet this is not always the case, and you can't be sure without inquiring to find out. All dentists need a license to practice, and to receive that they need to meet basic requirements that include an education requirement, a clinical requirement, and a written exam. The requirements for dental licensing vary by state, so you would need to check with your individual state to see what the requirements are there. Board certification is something dentists can choose to do beyond being licensed. It demonstrates an expertise, extensive experience, advanced training, technological advancement in the field, and a commitment to the dental field.

2. **Is there a particular area that the dentist specializes in?**
   This is an important question to ask so that you know what the dentist is spending most of their time on all week long. If you are looking for a dentist, for example, who does a lot of cosmetic dentistry, then you will want to pick one that has many years of experience in cosmetic dentistry. If they only see a few patients per year for cosmetic dentistry, then they will not have a lot of experience providing such treatments. Likewise, if you want a dentist who is child friendly, you want to ensure that the one you choose has many patients who are children, otherwise they won't have the experience you are looking for when it comes to treating children.

3. **What types of treatments are available at that dentist's office?**
   You would think that you could have just about any type of treatment you need, but that's not always the case. There are many dentists who do not offer particular treatments, such as veneers, crowns, or extractions. It's always a good idea to know what the depth of service is going to be like. If the dentist doesn't do much beyond fillings, then you will be referred to someone else every time treatment is needed.

4. **Are there some real-life photos of people they have provided treatment to?**
   Being able to see some before and after photos of some of the treatments they have provided to real-life people is huge. This will help you get an idea of what the dentist is capable of. Be sure you are not being shown stock photography photos, because those are not real people that the dentist has provided treatment to. You don't want to see the work that a stranger did, you want to see what this particular dentist can do. Those who have the experience and are proud of the work they have done will be happy to show you before and after photos.

5. **Do they have testimonials from happy patients?**
   Knowing that they have plenty of other satisfied patients can help bring you some comfort. Most dentist's offices that are worth their weight in gold can easily show you an array of testimonials. Be sure to read over the testimonials and see if the people were happy with their experience and what it is that they say they liked about the dentist and overall experience there. Don't feel like you have to stop at just reading the testimonials. There is nothing wrong with asking if they have a patient or two who you could speak with to inquire about their experience at the office.

6. **When asking about experience, ask about how many cases they have treated.**
   If you want to know how many crowns a dentist has done, for example, you are better off asking how many cases they have completed. This is because their answer if you are inquiring about how many crowns they have done may include numerous ones that were done on the same one patient. If you ask about cases, on the other hand, you will get a better idea of many different patients the dentist has provided that treatment to.

7. **How many years has the dentist been providing services?**
   While you want to know how long the person has been a dentist, you also should inquire about how long they have been providing specific treatments if you are interested in cosmetic dentistry, for example. If you know you need a porcelain veneer, you want to ask how many porcelain veneer cases they have completed and how long they have been providing the service.

8. **Does the dentist teach others and keep up on continuing education?**
   Education is an important part of the dental field, but it should continue once dental school is over. Some dentists provide teaching and educational opportunities to others in the field. It's also important that they keep up on continuing education so they know what is new and are aware of the advancements in the industry. You can narrow the focus of the question by asking what type of continuing education did they have in the last year or so.

9. **Which laboratory do they use if things like veneers are crowns are needed?**
   The quality of a porcelain veneer or crown is important and not something that should be ignored. There are plenty of labs that offer the services, and prices and quality vary widely. A quick online search of the lab they use can give you an idea if they use a quality one or not. Today there is a growing trend to use cheap dental labs in China and India. Many of these labs use substandard or even dangerous materials. You don't want your dentist cutting corners asking "How can we do this cheaper?" The quality and professionalism of the lab they use will have an impact on the quality of your treatment, should you need any of those services that call for lab work. You can always find it cheaper, but at what long-term cost. If your dental work needs replaced after a few years, did you really save any money?

10. How much are treatments and what type of payment options are available?

When you are asking this question, it helps if you already know on your end what your situation is. If you have dental insurance, you will want to know what it covers and how much you will be responsible for. Also, find out if it matters what dentist you go to, or if you have to choose from a particular list. If you have no dental insurance, inquire from the dental office what type of options they offer. Keep in mind that costs should not be your most important factor when choosing a dentist. It's great to know the information ahead of time, but it's never a good idea to choose a dentist based off of the price of treatments. When you are paying for a dental treatment, you are essentially paying for the dentist's expertise. You want a dentist who is well experienced and will provide the best, highest quality treatment. That's the main objective, not finding a dentist who has the lowest rates you can find.

11. Does the dentist check for things like oral cancer and correct bite?

There are many important issues when it comes to oral care, and you need a dentist who will keep up on all of it. You want to ensure that the office does things like screen for oral cancer, checks for decay and gum disease, and will also check to ensure that you have a correct bite. Without having a correct bite, your teeth can break, because of the stress, which makes it important that such things are considered.

These are 11 of the most important questions you will want to ask every dentist. By asking the right questions, you will get a deeper sense of what the dentist is capable of. These are things that may become a major issue later on if you don't know the answer to them from the start.

Most people don't take much effort in choosing the best dentist for them and their family. That's why they tend to go from dentist to dentist and end up with horror stories that they tell their friends. Problems that weren't treated correctly, issues that became worse, and more. Whether or not you like the treatment outcomes and your overall dental experience is going to come down to how much effort you put into finding the right dentist to begin with. You can avoid a lot of problems and headaches if you find the right dentist from the start.

If you are happy with your teeth, you will be happier in general. So don't count the questions, make the questions count.

CHAPTER 8
Why Not a Guarantee?

One of the questions you will want to ask any dentist you are considering is if they offer a guarantee. This is especially important if you are getting cosmetic dentistry or will be having treatments done. If they raise an eyebrow and think that it's a strange question, ask why they do not offer a guarantee. In our offices, we have always offered one and always will.

Offering our patients a guarantee on the treatments that we provide is a way of letting them know we absolutely stand behind our work. We are committed to making sure that it's to their satisfaction and if there's a problem we won't leave them hanging. We will be there with them to help make it right until they are satisfied. We see our relationship as a partnership, and we try to treat people like family. We wouldn't tell our family member that we are sorry they don't like the way it turned out and there's nothing that can be done. No, we would go to great lengths to help correct the problem, and it's the same thing we will do for every one of our patients.

The dentist you choose should be serious about standing behind their work.

But let's be honest, you may not get the response you want. You may be told there are no guarantees. In fact, you may be made to feel like it's out of the question to ask such a question. Don't be surprised if this happens to you at more than one dental office, but know that there are dentists out there who stand by their work and will offer a guarantee.

Health care is notorious for no guarantees.

Surgeons have a dark-humor insiders' joke: Dead patients can't sue.

If you've seen reality TV shows about plastic surgery, like the popular one called "BOTCHED," you know things can go horribly wrong. Guarantees are controversial in all kinds of health care including orthodontics. Many doctors are upset by the very idea. One huffed-and-puffed at me, "What do you think you're doing with this guarantee nonsense? We aren't operating Midas Muffler® shops, installing mufflers and guaranteeing them for 5,000 miles. We are doctors, dammit." His doctor-ego was mightily offended. But I doubt you will be, with the challenge of deciding who should be your family's trusted dentist. So, yes, I think there should be a guarantee! In fact, guarantees, plural!

The dentist you choose should offer some type of guarantee on the treatments that you will be having done. If they offer a guarantee, find out what it includes. Some may call it a warranty on the work as well, but again you want to know exactly what that means. There are some dentists who may offer a guarantee on their work, but it may also come with the stipulation that you remain a patient of theirs for five years after receiving the treatment.

You want to be well aware of the terms and conditions of the guarantee or warranty that they are offering, so you can see if it's legitimate or something they are trying to pass as being an honest backing of their work. Your dentist should want you to feel confident with the decision to have your treatment done at their office. If they provide high-quality care, then they should also offer a guarantee.

The Type of Guarantee

Typically, if the dentist is going to back the work they do, they will offer it on the services that they provide. These include such treatments as dental fillings, implants, crowns, and bridges. If they offer braces in their office, then they should also offer the same type of guarantee. When people get braces in my office, I want to make absolutely certain that they are happy with the outcome, and I guarantee to help them get there.

What people are generally protected against when it comes to dentist guarantees are breakage, loosening or detachment, or decay that may happen under the restoration. This is important to have, because the last thing you want is to put out $3,000 on two crowns only to have one break or fall off six months later. Without the dentist guaranteeing the work that they have done, where will that leave you? It would leave you shelling out more money to get it fixed. What if it doesn't last this time?

You simply can't put out the kind of money that it costs for dental treatments and not get some kind of guarantee that the dentist will be there to help make things right if something goes wrong. The average cost of a dental bridge is around $1,000 per tooth, and porcelain crowns can cost up to $3,000 per tooth. That's a significant investment you are making in your mouth, and you need some kind of guarantee that it's going to do what you are paying for.

You wouldn't go purchase a large screen television without the ability to have it replaced or repaired if three months later it stopped working. We don't spend that kind of money without trusting that we are going to be able to use it for a while and it's going to do what it's intended to do. The same concept holds true with dental work. If you pay for dental work, you should be able to trust that it's going to hold up for the amount of time that the dentist advised it would.

A guarantee from the dentist doesn't mean you can go be reckless with the tooth and run back and get it fixed. Dentists are going to provide you with instructions on how to care for the treatment that you had done, and in order to be eligible for the guarantee you are going to have live up to your end of the deal, by following their instructions and taking care of the teeth that had the treatments.

While you want the guarantee on the work, you also need to be aware that routine lifespan won't be covered. And that's a fair thing, and as it should be. You wouldn't expect to get a crown, for example, and assume that it will last you the rest of your life and if it doesn't that the dentist will fix it and have you on your way. The lifespan of a crown greatly varies. Some people may find that they last 10 years, but others may have one that lasts 30 years. Be sure to ask the dentist how long you can expect the work that is being performed to last. Having an honest assessment will let you know what to expect to get out of it in terms of lifespan.

Any dentist's office that believes in the quality of what they are doing will offer a guarantee of some kind. Knowing what that guarantee is and what is included is the best way to know how confident they are in their work and what you can expect if something were to go wrong. When you invest in your teeth, you want to feel confident and comfortable that you will get what you are paying for, and that it will be of high quality. This is something you want to know for every type of treatment that you may get at the dentist's office.

What Invalidates a Guarantee

If the dentist offers a guarantee, you want to know what will invalidate it as well. This information should be in written form so that you can keep the information and refer back to it. Not having it from the start opens the door to interpretation later that could cause issues. It's like playing a game without both sides being aware of what the rules are. Everyone needs to go into this knowing what the rules are. So find out what the guarantee is, and what types of things would invalidate it.

Of course, this will vary for every dentist who offers a guarantee, but it gives you an idea of what to watch for and inquire about. They include such things as:

- Not returning to the dentist for a routine check-up at least once a year during the period for which they guaranteed the work that was done. Most dentists who offer a guarantee will want you to keep up your end of good oral hygiene practices, which includes keep up with your preventive checkups.
- Not keeping up with your oral hygiene practices. Let's say that you go get some work done and then you decide you no longer feel like doing the work to keep up on brushing your teeth. I know it seems

crazy, but trust me, there are people who fall into lazy habits and they stop brushing or they get haphazard, only brushing periodically.

- Not following the instructions that the dentist provided for caring for the work that was done. If there is something specific that you were informed needed to be done to care for the work, then you will have to hold up your end of the bargain by following through with doing those tasks. The dentist will be clear about providing you with that information before the work is done, so that you are not blindsided with it later on.
- Accidents that may cause harm to the work that was done. What this means is that your husband doesn't get a bridge put in and then a couple of months later while playing on the men's basketball team he takes an elbow to the mouth while guarding a game-winning shot. If that elbow to the mouth breaks or damages the bridge, then it won't fall under the guarantee for the dentist to fix it free of charge.
- Illnesses that you may have or get that lead to damage in your teeth, gums or bones in the mouth. For example, if you have diabetes, epilepsy, or you undergo chemotherapy, it may have a negative effect on your dental condition. This is something that is beyond the scope of the work that the dentist provided, so it wouldn't be covered under the guarantee in most cases.

The guarantee that you get from a dentist isn't a free-for-all so that you can treat your teeth any old way you want and then head back into the office, expecting them to repair it under the guise of their guarantee. You want a guarantee that will cover the work that they did and their craftsmanship. You want the work to be of high quality, so that when you walk out the door you are confident that the bridge is going to hold up, or the fillings you just had put in are not going to fall apart or fall out a week later.

A dentist who is confident with the work that they do will offer some type of guarantee on it. They will stand behind what their treatments and they will be forthcoming in letting you know ahead of time what to expect, how to care for the work they have done, what the guarantee covers, and what your end of the arrangement is. This is fair, and this is a sign of a good dentist.

The amount of time that a dentist will guarantee the work for that they are doing also varies, but it's reasonable for you to find a five-year guarantee on a bridge or inlay, a three-year guarantee on ceramic veneers, three to four years on a combination treatment of a crown and bridge, a year on a full set of dentures, and a year on composite fillings. This gives you something to look for and ask about, so that you have the peace of mind for that time frame that the work they are providing will hold up on its own, without outside forces (such as accidents or neglect) causing problems.

Prevention Solutions

A dentist's office that provides a guarantee is one that shows they believe in a long term commitment to your dental health. They will also be forthcoming with the information on how to care for your teeth between dental visits, so that you can extend the life of any of your dental work, and you can help to have better oral hygiene and health all the way around. Much of the information they provide is geared toward prevention, as it should be.

Prevention is the best way to take care of our health, and the same goes for our oral health. When we take steps to take care of our teeth, gums, and overall oral health, we will be a better position to help avoid needing treatments in the first place. Preventative dentistry, which is caring for the teeth in order to help keep them healthy and prevent problems, should be high on everyone's priority list.

Many people focus on children when it comes to dental problems, but adults get plenty of them as well. It's imperative to maintain good dental hygiene practices all throughout your life, from childhood into old age, in order to help keep teeth healthy and lower the risks of getting other associated diseases that can stem from things like gum disease. By keeping up on your regular dental visits, you will be doing a world of good in helping to care for your overall dental health, as well as your general health.

If the dentists you interview for the position do not offer a guarantee, ask them why not. As someone who will be investing time and money, you deserve a guarantee that will help ensure you are receiving great treatment, and that the dentist stands behind the work that they do. Finding a dentist who guarantees the work that they do should not be difficult, but it is something that will help you weed through candidates in order to narrow down the list to the better ones.

You deserve a guarantee, and there is a great dentist out there who is ready to offer you one.

CHAPTER 9

How to Tackle the Ugly Matter of Money

You know it's coming and I know it's coming. We can't possibly have a discussion about dental work without having the discussion about, well, how it's going to be paid for. Like any other type of medical or health services, taking care of your teeth and oral health comes at a price. Granted, it's a smart investment and well worth making, but you still need the info how to get the bill paid for when the time comes.

Relax. This is an area where most people tend to focus too much and worry far more than they need to.

Yes, whatever work you have done going to the dentist is going to come with a bill, but that's to be expected. Depending on what services and treatments are being done, it could range from $100 for a cleaning and exam to thousands of dollars for braces. Still, there's no need to panic at this point.

You will be able to pay your dental tab without breaking the bank.

Whether or not you have dental insurance, you may still be paying for some of your bill out of pocket. Dental insurance doesn't usually pick up the tab for everything, so you should expect that you will be paying a portion. What portion becomes your responsibility will be determined by what procedures you have done. Some things cost more than others. For example, if you are merely going for a cleaning and exam that's not something costly and you won't need to take loans for it. But if you need several crowns or your child needs braces, that's going to be in the thousands and there's a good chance that you will need some payment options.

The good news is that payment options are usually available. Just about every dentist and orthodontist I've ever spoken to does offer some sort of payment options. They expect that patients will need the information, and so they usually have it ready for you when you need it. They have looked into the options that are available, have compiled the info, and can offer you what they know to be the best routes for you to consider. Of course you can go beyond that and do some research on your own, too, but what they are offering is a good starting place.

The first thing you will want to do is find out the specifics of your insurance policy, because that is going to have a lot to do with how much you end up paying out of pocket. Some insurance plans may pay for just about everything, while others may split the cost with you, or only pay a small portion. There are many different types of dental insurance plans out there, with each of them offering a variety of plans. One way that many people help pay for their dental bills is through using their benefits known as "flex spending," where an account through their job can be used to pay for dental bills through pre-tax dollars.

Avoiding Flex Spending Headaches
Some people find that flex spending arrangements are a headache and they may even try to avoid them, at times avoiding the dental work all together or paying for it another way. The good news is that there are ways that you can help to eliminate the flex spending headaches. It all comes down to knowing what to do to make it easier and avoid the stress that comes with such accounts if you don't plan ahead.

There are three main solutions you can take to get the most out of your employer's flex plan so that the amount out of your pocket   is reduced to a more manageable figure. Here are the three solutions you can start taking action with today:

1. **Sign up early.** Preparation is key to success in any endeavor. So make the most of your flex plan. Set aside your flex spending dollars now. Many employers set higher limits than you think on the amount of flex spending dollars you can contribute each year, tax free, from your salary to pay for health care expenses, such as dental care. Case in point: Many employers allow $2,500 or even $5,000 of pre-tax earnings to be set aside for your flex plan. Are you getting all of that money you can to pay for your family's dental care? You may not be. If you fail to sign up early, it could cost you more out-of -pocket for dental expenses, especially if your plan is not set up and ready before the treatment begins. If you have a new plan, work with your plan administrator to sign up early for next year in order to help maximize your savings.

2. **Make sure your employer is aware of any family status change.** Employers all have their own sign-up deadlines for flex plans, but typically at the beginning of the year, your employer asks you how much money you want to contribute to your flex plan for the year.

The problem with making annual decisions about your healthcare coverage is that you only have the opportunity to enroll, unless you have a qualified "family status change." What exactly is a family status change? They are things like marriage, divorce, births, and a loss of a spouse's insurance coverage. Each of these status changes are qualified reasons to change your plan, and possibly add more coverage for dental care, yet most people are not aware of it.

3. **Choose wisely.** Finally, give some thought to calculating how much money to contribute to your flex plan at work this year. If you are considering some cosmetic dentistry or orthodontic treatments, visit your doctor's offices for the initial consultation. Their office can help you plan exactly how much money you should contribute to help reduce your out-of-pocket expenses when it's time to pay for, and receive, the procedure you are inquiring about.

Here's something you may not know about your flex plan: If you put in more money than you need, by law, you lose the money. You have three months after the end of the calendar year to submit claims for eligible expenses from the previous calendar year. Any money left in your account after this three-month period is lost.

The Scoop on Insurance

I can tell you that today there are as many different types of insurance as there are patients. And every one of them tends to be a bit different, all offering something unique, and paying for different things in varying amounts. I can't possibly speak to your specific and unique insurance policy without seeing it first, but I can say that in general and in my experience, most dental insurance is going to cover some of your expenses beyond a yearly exam and cleaning. What amount they cover is going to be the part that varies, and will be information you will want to know ahead of time.

If you don't have dental insurance, or you would like to make a switch to find a better plan, you are in luck. There are many dental insurance plans and they are often quite affordable. Some of the different types of dental insurance plans that are offered include:

• Table or schedule of allowance plans. These plans have a pre-determined list of treatments and what they will pay for each of them. The information stays consistent regardless of where you go for treatment. Whatever the difference is between what they will pay for the treatment and what the dentist bills you for it would be your responsibility to pay. Unless you have a secondary insurance plan to pick up that extra, you will be paying that out-of-pocket.

• Direct reimbursement programs. This type of dental insurance plan comes with a pre-determined amount or percentage that the company will pay toward your dental care. With this type of plan, you can usually go to the dentist of your choice. They may say, for example, that they will pay 50% of the bill on all of your crowns, veneers, or bridges. If this is the case, you may want to work with the dentist to get the best possible rate, since it will save you from paying more out of your own pocket.

• UCR plans, which stands for "usual, customary, and reasonable," which is a plan that will pay a usual, customary, or reasonable fee to the dentist for the services rendered. The patient can usually choose which dentist they want to go to as well. With this type of plan, the insurance company has a payment agreement with the dentist's office.

Again, dental insurance plans vary, so you have to choose the one that is going to be the best for your family. Know what it covers and what is expected of you. Find out if it requires you go to a specific dentist's office, or if you can choose your own dentist. You want to be able to choose your own dentist, because you can't possibly find the best dentist for your family by letting someone else make that decision for you (especially allowing an insurance company to make that decision for you).

Never let money keep you from having good oral health. It's too important to overlook and skip it.

CHAPTER 10

Is Sedation Dentistry a Good Idea?

Every year around the country, there are millions of people who have such fear of going to the dentist that they just skip it. Yes, the fear of all the what ifs and what could happens consumes them to the point that they literally don't ever go to the dentist. This is the case whether they are in pain or they simply need a routine cleaning. They continue to avoid the dentist, allowing the fear and anxiety to rule supreme.

Meanwhile, what happens is that their teeth end up having more and more problems. If you are someone who avoids going to the dentist out of fear, there is a good chance that you will end up having more oral health problems. And as we know from previous chapters, poor oral health can increase chances of poor overall health. So what is it exactly that creates this heightened sense of fear regarding to the dentist, and what can be done about it? That's the important question that everyone who has experienced this or who has a loved one who needs information so that they can overcome this problem.

We must remember that our overall health is tied to our oral health.

The more we understand the problem of fear and anxiety that people have for going to the dentist, the more we will be able to tackle the problem. Without addressing it, those who have the fear will likely suffer from poor oral health. Plus, our smile says a lot about us. What happens if you always avoid the dentist? What can a smile that never goes the dentist say about the person? There is a good chance they will not have the smile and teeth they wish they did, and it will hold them back from a lot of things. They will tend to be less confident and may avoid many social situations as a result.

Why People Have Dental Fear and Anxiety

For the millions of people who have an extreme fear of going to the dentist, the reasons why may vary as much as the people themselves. There is no one definitive reason why someone has such anxiety about going to the dentist that it prompts them to literally feel sick and avoid it at all costs. Some people have such anxiety about the dentist because of childhood experiences gone wrong. When they were a child, they may have gone to a dentist who scared or hurt them, and it created a lasting image that made them fearful to ever go back to another one.

This is one of the reasons why it is so important to find the right dentist for your family. We all know how important first impressions are, and you don't get a second chance to make a first impression. If a child goes to a dentist and it's not a good experience for them, then there is a good chance that will set the tone for future visits. They will become fearful and try to avoid going to the dentist. There are some people who are able to overcome this, often because their next experience with a different dentist was able to change their image and mindset, but that's not always the case. More often than not, if a child has a poor dental experience while they are young, they will grow up to think poorly about going to the dentist as an adult. If the experience was really bad, they may end up being one of the millions of people who at the mere thought of going for an appointment end up with anxiety, feeling sick, or becoming so upset that they literally can't go to the appointment.

Other factors that can contribute to people being overly fearful of going to the dentist include hearing other people's horror stories or watching videos and movies. There are videos and movies that put dental horror stories out there into the mainstream, and it can give people a lot of reason to be afraid to step foot into an dentist office. Still others may have a gag reflex that makes them afraid to go to the dentist. When they have their mouth open and work is being done, they may continuously and unintentionally gag. They fear they are going to choke, and this can cause some serious anxiety about being in the dental chair.

It's estimated that up to 15% of people in the country have fear and anxiety to the point that they avoid seeing the dentist.

Some people may suffer from anxiety about going to the dentist and some may have a phobia. We all experience some anxiety at times, as it can be a normal part of life. Some anxiety is even good for us, because it helps make us more alert and cautious in life and can help protect us. Those with anxiety about going to the dentist may feel nervous about their appointment, but many will still go to it. Those with a phobia regarding going to the dentist will avoid it at all costs. They believe they will be in real danger if they attend the appointment. It's an irrational fear about going when there is no real danger.

Those with a phobia about going to the dentist may experience panic, fear, a rapid heartbeat, shortness of breath, trembling, and an intense desire to get away. Their fight or flight instincts have told them there is danger and they need to get the heck out of dodge in order to protect themselves. Dodge, in this case, just so happens to be the dentist's office.

Other people who may consider using sedation dentistry are those who have difficulty sitting still. There are many people who have hyperactivity disorders and it is very difficult for them to sit still, especially for the amount of time that it may take to complete a procedure. Those who also have a low threshold for pain or who have very sensitive teeth may consider sedation dentistry. Both of these conditions could add to the fear and anxiety they experience at the dentist. Additionally, if there is someone who has a lot of work that needs to be done, they may be able to get more of it done at once by using sedation dentistry techniques. This could help cut down on the number of appointments that they need to go to in order to get all the work completed.

Whether you or someone in your family have an intense anxiety or phobia about going to the dentist, it's important to find ways to overcome that. Your oral health is too important to ignore because of an irrational fear. The good news is that with today's technology there are ways to help people move past their fears so that they can go to the dentist and still have great oral health.

Dental Sedation

An option that many people consider when it comes to being fearful of going to the dentist is sedation dentistry. It has become popular in recent years with both children and adults. Many people see it as the answer to help those who fear the dentist to be able to get past the fear and get the dental treatment that they need. But is it a good idea to opt for sedation dentistry? You can only answer that question when you know what it is, what all it involves, and what the alternatives may be.

Sedation dentistry, sometimes referred to as sleep dentistry, is the use of medication in order to help patients relax and move past their fear and anxiety. It's been around for a long time, but in recent years there have been many dentists who are promoting it, and many patients who are jumping at the chance to check it out and see if it helps them be able to get the appointment over without all the fear and anxiety. The medications that are used give the patient the ability to overcome the fear, without them having to try to do it all on their own. Left to try and overcome the fear on their own, many would never be able to do it.

There are various types of sedation dentistry, so it is important if you are considering it to speak with the dentist about which ones their office offers. These include:

- **Oral sedation** – This involves the patient taking a pill, usually about an hour before their appointment, then having someone else drive them to the dentist's office. Once there, they will be taken into care of the dental staff, who will see them through the appointment. The sedation keeps the person awake, but helps them to relax and be more comfortable throughout the appointment. Following the appointment, the patient would need to be driven home by someone else.
- **Nitrous oxide** – Otherwise known as "laughing gas," this type of sedation is administered by placing a mask over the nose. The person would breathe in the nitrous oxide, which would help them to relax and have a more comfortable experience through the appointment. If the inhaled sedation is minimal, the person may be able to drive themselves home.
- **IV sedation** – This type of sedation administers the drug through an IV, so it works faster. The dentist can also adjust the amount that is being administered to the patient as the appointment goes along.
- General anesthetic – With this practice, the patient is not awake during the procedure.

Sedation can range, being minimal, moderate, or deep, as well as the person being completely unconscious while under general anesthesia. Depending on the one that the person opts for, this will determine whether or not they are able to drive home on their own or if they need someone to do the driving for them. In addition to the sedation, a local anesthesia is still used in the mouth where the work will be performed. The local anesthesia is to keep the patient from feeling pain when the work is being done.

When considering whether or not sedation dentistry is a good idea for you, it's always wise to weigh the pros and cons and consider the alternative options. It can be a great way to help those who have anxiety and phobias be able to get the dental work done that they need, and to help them keep up with good oral health. The medications used for oral sedation are considered safe, and they have been found to be very effective in helping people to relax so they can get their dental work done.

There are a few downsides to using some of the particular mediations, which include that they can take a while to be effective. This means that, depending on when it was taken, it may not yet be effective when the appointment time comes. Also, it could be challenging to determine the best dosage that someone should take in order to achieve the desired results, and they can't usually be adjusted once the procedure is underway. There is also a limit to how much can be taken, so if someone needs more than what is allowed they may not be able to get the effect that is needed in order to have a comfortable appointment. Also, some of the medications can create a type of hangover, which will leave people feeling a little spaced out, and it can last for even a couple of days.

When it comes to children, there are dentists who offer sedation dentistry. The American Academy of Pediatrics recommends that parents have thorough knowledge about the sedation and what to expect, so that they can help their child through the process to help ensure a successful outcome. Their recommendation is that parents can help children to prepare for the appointment, know what to do during the appointment, and after it is over. They offer detailed guidelines for parents on their website. Sedation dentistry use on children is controversial, as there are some people on both sides of the issue, with some for and against the use of it. If you are considering using sedation dentistry on your child, speak with the dentist, as well as your pediatrician, to get opinions and recommendations.

The costs of sedation dentistry vary, depending on the type you will be getting. They range from around $50 for nitrous oxide to $250 for oral sedation to around $600 for IV sedation.

Not every dentist's office will offer these types of sedation dentistry. Some of the types of sedation require training and that emergency supplies be on hand. Most states require that the dentist have a license to offer sedation dentistry, so you will need to inquire about what types the particular dentist you are considering going to offers. If you are going to have sedation dentistry done, you want to make sure you are with a dentist who is well experienced and qualified in providing it. The license required to administer sedation dentistry is determined by the dental board in your state. You have the ability to inquire with them about what is required in your state.

If you have health conditions, such as diabetes, cardiac conditions, hypertension, or other serious issues, be sure to speak with your physician about sedation dentistry if you are considering having it done. It's always a good idea to get their approval to go ahead with it, as they will be more familiar with your overall health and know if you are a good candidate for it or not.

What the Science Says and the Alternatives

Over the years, there have been studies that focused on sedation dentistry. This is always a good thing, because it provides us with a little something to back up the ideas behind the practice. In the April 2016 issue of the journal Dental Clinics of North America, they report that orally administered sedation is useful for treatment of anxious adults and pediatrics patients. They state that it is a cost-effective and effective service that is widely available, and it enables the dentist to provide care to millions who would otherwise have their dental needs unmet.

The Centers for Disease Control and Prevention reports that almost 19% of children and nearly 32% of adults have untreated dental caries at any given time. This means that millions of children and adults are walking around with cavities in their mouth that are being left untreated. If some of those are due to fear and anxiety over going to the dentist, and millions of them would have to be, then sedation dentistry is going to provide a good option for them to consider. There can be some terrible consequences to not getting dental work done, which makes sedation dentistry a solution that should be considered for those who would otherwise go without getting the work done at all.

For those who have concerns about sedation dentistry and want to explore alternatives to overcoming the anxiety or phobia, there are options. One of the most important things you can do for your family in order to overcome dental anxiety is to find the right dentist to begin with. The right dentist will be the first step in helping to put the person at ease and make them feel comfortable. They will be understanding of their fears and anxiety and help to alleviate it, as well as offer options for overcoming it, including ones that don't involve sedation dentistry.

It's important for those who have anxiety and phobias about the dentist to recognize that is what it is, and to talk about it. When they discuss it with their dentist, they may discover ways to work through it, so that the dental work can still be done. The patient can also work through it by starting with short and easy appointments, and work their way up to ones that require more work. This way they will feel more comfortable with each visit. They may also be more comfortable if they can bring a trusted person with them to the appointment, so that it helps to calm them down and feel safer.

Additionally, it's a good idea for the person to learn distraction methods, so that they are not focused on thinking about the dentist's appointment, and to learn relaxation techniques. Using something like a television show or headphones will help to distract the patient while work is being performed. Relaxation techniques, which can be useful in many situations in life, can help to immediately relax people. They include focusing on breathing, where your attention is turned to just focusing on the breath. This is a type of mediation that helps to calm you down. Also, using a visualization technique can be helpful, as the person keeps their mind focused on something positive that they enjoy, such relaxing at the beach.

Those who have a serious phobia regarding going to the dentist may benefit from speaking with a psychologist. They can help the person to work through the problem and possibly move past it so that they can become more comfortable going to the dentist.

Making the Call

So, we are brought back to our original question: Is sedation dentistry a good idea? The bottom line regarding it is that yes, for many people it is a good idea. There are some people who would otherwise not get the dental treatment they need without having the option of using sedation dentistry. For that reason alone, it stands to reason that sedation dentistry is a good option for many people.

Whether or not it is the right option for your family depends on the factors involved, including the level of fear and anxiety present, how their overall health is, and what their doctor recommendation would be. Also, it's important to make sure that if you are considering it, you speak to the dentist and get all the details regarding what to do beforehand, what to expect during it, and what will happen once it is over. Only when you have all the information can you make an informed decision that will be the right one for you and your family.

Finding the right dentist is essential, especially if you are considering sedation dentistry. It's an area that plays an important role for millions of people, and one that the dentist needs to be experienced and knowledgeable about. Only you will know if choosing sedation dentistry is the right route, but at least now you know more about it and can use this information in helping to make your decision.

CHAPTER 11

Creating Smiles by Design: Cosmetic Dentistry

One of the reasons that I named my practice "Smiles by Design" is because I see dentistry as a design process of beautification, and the end result - a healthy, bright smile - as a work of art.

Helping patients achieve smiles that they are proud of and that helps them feel good about themselves is one of the most rewarding things about this profession. We are proud to offer various cosmetic dentistry services and "smile makeovers" that will keep you smiling for many years to come!

What is Cosmetic Dentistry?

There are millions of people each year who opt for cosmetic dentistry. This is because cosmetic dentistry can be a great way to enhance your appearance, as well as compliment your overall health, and help to maintain your oral health. Cosmetic dentistry can help you improve tooth function, as well as help you love your smile.

There are numerous procedures that are included under the umbrella of cosmetic dentistry. Some of these procedures include bonding, implants, bridges, dentures, braces, periodontal plastic surgery, crowns, veneers, teeth whitening, and tooth-colored fillings. There are many options available, and each depends on what you may need and what your overall oral health goals may be. You may be a good candidate for some these procedures, but it's always good to discuss it with your trusted dentist. This is one more reminder why it is so important to have the best dentist for you. It's important that you have complete trust in your dentist and that you feel they will be making the best recommendations for you and putting your best interests ahead.

Let's look at a few of these popular common cosmetic dentistry options that are available today.

Porcelain crowns. A solid choice for those who have a damaged tooth, porcelain crowns are made to fit over the damaged tooth, down to the gum. It provides a strong and resilient tooth covering that looks natural and functions like your regular tooth. Those who get large fillings may be a good option for getting porcelain crown inlays or onlays. The inlays are porcelain that is put over the grooves and cusp tip, while the onlays are often used to give a new look to an old filling. The porcelain color can be made to match the color of the tooth, helping to provide a natural look.

Porcelain veneers. Creating a natural smile is easier when you opt for procedures such as porcelain veneers. Again, porcelain provides strength and durability, while helping to create a natural look. Thin pieces of porcelain are used to replace your original tooth enamel. They adhere right to the tooth, giving your tooth a nice, natural look and natural function. To put them on, a tiny amount of enamel from the tooth is removed. They are a popular option for those who may have a discolored tooth or have issues with the shape of their tooth, as well as those who have overlaps or small gaps. With veneers, your own teeth stay intact for the most part, and they resist stains from such things as coffee, tea, and smoking cigarettes. The one drawback that you need to be aware of when considering porcelain veneers is that it is not considered reversible, because a tiny amount of enamel on the teeth was removed in order to put them on.

Bonding. Bonding is a popular option that involves a filling material that is attached to the original tooth. This is an ideal option for those who have a chipped or broken tooth, or someone who has a tooth that is improperly shaped. For those who have a tooth that is peg-shaped or smaller than it should be, this is a good option to consider. The filling material is bonded to the original tooth enamel and dentin, so that it looks and feels natural. It also functions like your regular tooth, so you will feel comfortable with using the tooth that has bonding. Tooth bonding is a procedure that offers a great way to help repair chipped teeth or address other issues.

Dentures. There are several options when it comes to dentures, including partial dentures, full dentures, and overdentures. Some forms of dentures have been used for many years. Depending on how many teeth are missing or the types of gum conditions that someone may have, dentures may be a good option. Partial dentures are used when someone is missing groups of teeth, while full dentures are used to replace both teeth and gums. Overdentures are a newer option in the world of dentures. The process of using overdentures involves having implants put in that help to keep the denture in place. It's believed that overdentures may also help with better long-term success, because it may help eliminate bone loss where the implants are located.

Porcelain fixed bridges. Porcelain options are a popular choice in cosmetic dentistry. They offer durability and they look great, making more people feel comfortable having them. A porcelain fixed bridge is an option that is available for someone who is missing one or more teeth. The porcelain fixed bridge is created to look just like the natural tooth that it is replacing, usually creating a flawless look to a problem area. It's a popular option to consider for those who are missing teeth or who have teeth that are damaged.

Tooth-colored fillings. Years ago, people got metal fillings. Today there are millions of people who have several metal fillings in their mouth. Often times they need to be replaced over time, and other times people want a better look. Rather than opening their mouth to laugh and showing their metal fillings, they are opting for tooth-colored fillings. Whether you are getting a filling for the first time, are replacing an old one that is worn out, or you want to enhance your look, tooth-colored fillings are an ideal choice. The composite resins and porcelains that are used today for fillings help to keep the metal out of the mouth and provide a more natural look and feel.

Teeth whitening. Nobody wants to have a smile that shows teeth stained from coffee, tea, or cigarette smoking, among other things. There are plenty of options available today for whitening your teeth, which will give you the confidence you want and need, and help create a more beautiful smile. While there are products available in the stores, they will never compare in quality to what your dentist can offer. Teeth whitening is an affordable cosmetic dentistry option for those who want to enhance their look. There are several types of dentist-provided teeth whitening options available today, including both in-office and at-home approaches. In-office teeth whitening will focus on using a stronger whitening agent, while still protecting the tooth. In just one visit, you can see a difference in the color of your teeth, often brightening several shades with just one application. Depending on how well you take care of your teeth, the whitening that you have done can last for a year or even several years before needing it done again to maintain your brighter smile. Your dentist can provide you with such things as custom fitted mouth trays for whitening your teeth, which will give you a more successful whitening. Most people believe that whiter teeth are more appealing, which makes teeth whitening one of the most common cosmetic dentistry options there is. It's usually an option that is affordable, easy to do, provides good results, and one that helps people love their smile and feel more confident showing it off.

Braces. Braces can be both cosmetic and a medical necessity. You are going to have a perfect smile, and you will avoid problems that misaligned teeth can cause. No longer just for pre-teens, there are millions of adults even getting braces today. Not only are they a great way to help give you the beautiful smile that you want, but they will help protect your overall oral health by addressing problems. While traditional metal braces are available, there are other more discreet options available today, including clear aligners that you can take out for an hour per day in order to eat and brush your teeth. The field has come a long way in terms of straightening teeth, and you may find that you want to get the braces that you should have had a couple of decades ago.

There are numerous options available today in cosmetic dentistry. If you have issues that you want addressed, you should explore your options. Speak with the dentist to see if they feel it is also a good fit for your situation, and explore all of the options that they offer at that office. As technology continuously changes, new procedures emerge. Even if there isn't an option that appeals to you today, there is a good chance that one may appeal to you in the near future. Like other areas in life, the dental industry is always changing, as we look for ways to improve people's lives through good oral health and a beautiful smile.

Making the Decision

When it comes to whether or not cosmetic dentistry is the right fit for you and your family, you have a few things to consider.

For starters, what your overall goals are in getting it done. Consider whether or not it's going to add a better quality of life, help protect your overall health, or if it will be beneficial in other ways.

Your teeth are such an important part of your life, your character, and in your overall health, that considering cosmetic or implant dentistry makes good sense. If you are someone who is missing teeth, has worn-out crowns, has a chipped tooth, wants to replace metal crowns, or would like to have teeth that just look better, there is an option for you. Today's cosmetic dentistry field is high-tech, advanced, and provides many options that will give you a beautiful smile that looks and feels natural. It will help you get the most out of your teeth for the long haul, and help to protect your overall health and confidence level.

Increasingly there are insurance companies that are paying for cosmetic dentistry and implant options. They realize that there are many benefits to people getting the procedures done. If you are concerned about the costs associated with cosmetic dentistry, be sure to check with your insurance provider first to see what is covered and what options they offer, and speak with the dentist to see what options they can recommend.

Remember, getting dental work done may be seen as expensive, but it pales in comparison to the expense of not getting the work done.

Finding the right dentist for you so that you get the best treatment is essential. Make it a priority and your dental needs will be met in a way that keeps you smiling for many years to come.

CHAPTER 12

Implants and Implant Supported Dentures

Despite numerous improvements in dental care in the last several years, there are millions of people who are walking around with missing teeth. No, there really are. As we have discussed in prior chapters, there are many people who have dental problems which they do not have addressed. Dental issues are not a problem which you can ignore and expect it to just go away, and this very often leads to partial or even complete tooth loss. Often times, people will continue to leave them like that even after this has occurred.

We know that when you are missing teeth it can have devastating consequences. Those who are missing teeth tend to not be confident, because they know it doesn't look the best. They may end up hiding their mouth when they speak or laugh, and they may shy away from being in social groups. Teeth are something that people always look at in another person, and they help to give someone personality. One's teeth are their signature, if you will, or their unique fingerprint. Everyone has their own unique set of teeth and it helps to create who you are and what you look like.

When teeth are missing, there are going to be other problems even beyond the confidence issue. There can be health problems that arise as well. Teeth work together in what I like to think of as a team atmosphere. They all work together to give you the set of teeth you have. When there is one or more missing, there will be more of a strain or stress put on the others. The teeth next to where the open space is often shift to accommodate for the empty space. This can be devastating to the entire row of teeth, because it creates a dominoes-like shift in the mouth.

If you are someone who is missing teeth, or someone in your family is, what should you do? Is it best for you to continue ignoring it or just getting by, or is there a better route? Well, I'm glad you asked, because there is certainly a better route. The more you learn about the options available to help address a missing tooth, the better prepared you will be to get the situation taken care of. **In this chapter, we will explore the options that are out there for you: implant dentistry.**

What is Implant Dentistry?

For many years, the only treatment option for someone who is missing teeth was to get bridges or dentures. However, implant dentistry has become increasingly popular in recent years. It's important to know all you can about it if you will be considering it as an option for you or someone in your family. Implant dentistry helps people obtain a fuller, more natural-looking smile and it offers some other benefits as well.

Implant dentistry started in Sweden, when a team led by Dr. P.I. Branemark learned that titanium can bond with bone. Implant dentistry involves using a small threaded screw that is made out of titanium. The screw is implanted into your gum where your missing tooth is, and a crown is put over the end of the implant, which looks like your natural tooth and fits in with your other teeth. If you have a missing tooth and you don't have anything there to continue to stabilize the bone, it will lead to more damage. The bone that holds your teeth in place is essentially dissolved away once you lose a tooth. This can create a shift in your teeth and lead to additional tooth loss and gum problems.

When that happens, it can lead to problems with everything from your bite and how you chew to your facial appearance. Once your teeth begin to shift, it can have a dramatic impact on how you look. It can even impact how you speak. Some people who experience this go on to become withdrawn, because they are so embarrassed by what has happened and how they look, and they also end up having health problems due to poor nutrition. The shift and loss of teeth can have a detrimental effect on what people eat, thus leading to a poor diet.

Today, the success rate is around 96%, making the implants a great choice for most people. There are a few factors that need to be considered before opting for dental implants. It is believed that doctors who do more implants each year have a higher success rate, which stands to reason. Therefore, it's important to choose a dentist who is well experienced in doing implants. You want one who does over 50 implants per year, so that you will have a higher success rate from their being experienced.

Another factor that will be considered is the person's bone quality. The dentist will need to implant the screw into the bone, so there needs to be a minimal amount there in order to perform the procedure. This doesn't mean that if you already have bone loss there that it's too late for implants. Through sophisticated procedures, well experienced dentists can perform bone grafting in order to help you have the bone needed for the procedure. Typically, the bone would come from your own lower jaw, or it can even be taken from other sources, such as bovine bone or cadavers.

If you are considering having implants done, the dentist is going to need to know your medical history. A clinical exam and thorough medical history will be taken, so that they can be sure that you don't have any conditions that would create complications for the implants or for the medical conditions you have. Some of the medical problems that could be of concern include liver disease, diabetes, and bleeding disorders. If you have any of these conditions and are still interested in implant dentistry, speak with your trusted dentist. That's the only way to find out if it's a good fit for you or if there are better options with the conditions that you have.

With implants, there is a healing phase that can take months. During that time, you will wear a partial or full denture, so you will still be comfortable and your mouth will be fully functioning. Once your implants are finished and healed, it's important to continue to take

CROWN

ABUTMENT

SCREW

good care of them, just as you would your own natural teeth. Just like your natural teeth, they can develop bone loss, as well as gingivitis. You will need to brush and floss them daily, just as your natural teeth, as well as go for regular cleanings and exams. The implant offers a long-term solution that lasts for many years, and it will help you to maintain your jaw bone, which is a huge benefit in protecting your overall oral and general health.

There are some dentists who offer implant dentistry. If they do, it's a service that requires additional training in order to provide it. Many people go to a specialist for implants, such as a periodontist, or oral and maxillofacial surgeons. In choosing where to have yours done, be sure that the office is well experienced and is qualified to be offering the service. You can expect to pay around $3,000 or more per tooth, which doesn't include additional fees if you need bone grafting or the crown that will go on the titanium screw. Although you want to be aware of the average cost, the cost shouldn't be the most important factor. You must have a credentialed doctor perform the work, so make that your highest priority when deciding who will do it. You want quality work by a well experienced dentist, not the cheapest price you can find. There is a lot at stake, and it needs to be done right in order for you to have long-term success.

Implant Supported Dentures
You may be familiar with the fact that dental implants can act as an real, life-like replacement for a tooth, and they are definitely of great benefits to someone who still has many of their natural teeth.

However, what about if you are missing multiple teeth? Or you are missing multiple teeth in both jaws?

As an alternative to implants, some patients who are in these situations are great candidates for implant supported dentures. This is a middle ground between traditional dentures and implants, and one that tends to be more economically feasible than having a number of implants put in. Instead of using adhesive like dentures do, this method affords additional support by being secured with advanced full-arch dental implants. It is a low maintenance and effective method of smile correction that is popular among patients who have experienced tooth loss.

Loose dentures are not only uncomfortable, but they can make one feel self-conscious, as there is a fear of the denture slipping or falling out when a person wearing them is trying to eat or speak. This happens most often with the lower denture which can be easily dislodged by the tongue.

In addition to being uncomfortable, the constant removal, movement and adjustment of a denture can also cause bone loss in the jaw over a period of time, as a denture presses down on the ridges where your teeth were formerly supported.

Implant-supported dentures are a great option for individuals who are seeking an affordable option to significantly improve their ability to chew and smile. The support of the implant allows the dental fixture to be shaped into a horseshoe, reducing the bulkiness and opening the palate to create more space for the tongue and better ability to taste food. Implant-supported dentures are sturdier and do not require adhesive.

The individual can improve their diet by including fruits, veggies, steaks, corn on the cob, and other foods one would typically have to avoid with traditional dentures. Also, implant-supported dentures significantly improve patients' confidence to smile and speak.

This type of dentures is removable, and you'll be able to snap it on and off as many times as needed. This means that cleaning and maintaining the denture is just as easy as a traditional denture.

Benefits of Implant-Supported Dentures

Cost effectiveness is just one of several reasons why patients choose this method of smile correction. Implant supported dentures function more like natural teeth, thus restoring the patient's ability to chew foods that were previously off limits. They are also easy to clean as there is no adhesive needed for security, and the device is removable.

This option also preserves a patient's natural gum tissue and bone, making it overall more comfortable than other methods of tooth replacement.

The process of having implant supported dentures is fairly simple and pain free - essentially, the existing denture becomes the interim denture after the implant surgery. Several months after the surgery, the patient is provided a permanent denture device that snaps on to their implants. The process is simple and includes a series of appointments with our office to ensure that everything fits properly and to ensure that the patient is comfortable with their new appliance.

CHAPTER 13
Choose a Highly Successful Dentist

By this point, you know that choosing the right dentist for you and your family is crucial. There is a lot at stake, and you don't want to get it wrong. Far too often, people don't pay much attention to which dentist they choose, only to be disappointed once they have an appointment or two. Treat choosing a dentist as something highly important, because believe me, it is. It's more important than most people tend to realize, and it can have far-reaching consequences if you don't get it right.

Not having the right dentist at your side can lead to host of problems, many of which we have covered in this book. If you are with the wrong dentist, it can make you and your family want to back away from getting the treatment that they need. Appointments may be skipped, dreaded, or you may have anxiety about each one, making it difficult for to keep up with the routine. When it comes to your kids, you are creating a foundation for the relationship they will likely forever have with the dental world. The choices you make today could set them up to either fear and avoid going to the dentist later in life, or it could help them become more comfortable and feel that it's an important part of their overall health.

We already know there are devastating consequences to having poor oral health. When people have poor oral health, it affects their mental health, as well as their physical health. Children who have a poor oral health image will usually suffer from an increase in being bullied, a higher suicide rate, and they become more withdrawn. It can make them not want to participate in social interactions and even refrain from participating in school as they should.

Adults who have poor oral health can go on to have poor general health. There will also be social problems because of the dental image issues, including that they are more embarrassed, less confident, and may even get passed over for jobs and promotions. Those who don't care for their teeth or smile will usually try to hide it when they laugh or talk, making it difficult for them to participate in social interactions as they would like to. It can also have devastating effects on being able to find dates and romantic partners.

There are many great reasons for making your oral health a huge priority in your life, and not one good reason not to.

Just about every parent wants to help give their child the best start in life that they can. We want to protect them, help them learn to do the right thing, take good care of their health, and go on to become productive and successful adults. One thing we can do in helping us achieve those goals is to ensure that their dental needs are successfully met, so that they don't ever experience the life-changing problems that can arise from them not liking their teeth or smile.

As parents, we owe it to our children to help protect their teeth by ensuring they have the best dentist in their court. When they have a great dentist at their side, they will feel more comfortable knowing that the recommendations, treatments, and steps taken are in the best interest of the child. Children aside, you also deserve to have a great dentist. While I don't know what you have personally been through in your life when it comes to your dental experience, I can say without a doubt that I have come in contact with thousands of patients in my life. I have seen and heard it all, and I have also fixed it all, often times fixing what wasn't done right elsewhere.

When you find the right dentist, you will know it. You will have no doubt about it. You will feel it and you will no longer question whether you should continue on or look for another. Once you have the right dentist you come to have a sense of trust, and being in anyone else's chair simply won't do. Any other dentist you ever meet will be measured up against that one that you know is different, stands out, and is highly successful.

Your mission is to find a dentist who is highly successful. And if you choose to accept that mission, you will be successful at it.

Defining Highly Successful

To some extent, you could say that every dentist is successful. After all, they did go through dental school and they have succeeded in becoming a dentist in the first place. But that's about where it ends. Everything beyond that is going to be what separates those who simply made it as a dentist and those who have gone on to become highly successful dentists. As you can imagine, there are going to be a lot fewer highly successful dentists out there than there are simply dentists.

Many people who finish dental school either get a job in someone else's office or they hang out their own shingle to open their practice. This puts them in business and they can start seeing patients. But that doesn't mean at all that they are a great dentist, that they have the experience you want or need, or that they even care about being highly successful.

In fact, I can tell you that many dentists don't give a rat's behind about being highly successful. They simply want to clock in at 9 each day and clock out at 5 to go home, and they don't care much about what goes on between those hours. Sure, they want to put forth the effort to perform treatments for their patients, but they won't even raise an eyebrow if they lose patients. That's because, to be honest with you, they don't do much to keep those patients in the first place. My guess is you have been to a dentist or even two who was just like this.

For starters, let me tell you what a good dentist is like. A good dentist will meet your needs when you go, and give you exactly what you expected. That good dentist will do exactly what you assumed would be done and treat you exactly how you thought you would or should be treated. And then there won't be much more beyond that. They don't feel they need to do anything else beyond that. After all, they are a good dentist and the patients seem to be satisfied and continue to come back.

Now let me tell you what it's like when you see a highly successful dentist. They won't stop at just meeting your needs. They know that meeting your needs and giving you what you expect should be the minimum that you get when you go to the dentist. When you go the office of a highly successful dentist, you will find that the bare minimum or just meeting your expectations will never do. They will always strive for more and will always go above and beyond. At their office, they want to know your name, the things you care about, they want to create a relationship with you, and they want you walking out feeling like you were a star visiting their office that day. They treat everyone like gold, because they realize how important every patient is. They want you to feel special and they will always, always go out of their way to treat you like they would treat their own family.

How's that for exceptional dental care?

Why would ever want to go do a dentist's office that just meets your expectations? Of course they should do that. They don't have to do much in order to meet your expectations, so they are not putting forth much effort. You deserve going to a dentist's office where they will always thumb their nose at the idea of just meeting expectations. You want the red carpet treatment, you want to feel like you belong there, and you want to feel understood and listened to. You want all of your questions answered about treatments and procedures, and you don't want the dentist keeping one eye on the clock as those questions are being answered.

Believe it or not, there are highly successful dentists out there, and one of them is waiting for you to become their patient. You didn't realize they exist, but now that you do, it should become a priority to find one for you and your family. You will love the difference that each appointment makes in how you feel when you have a highly successful dentist who genuinely cares about the patients, their best needs, rises above just meeting expectations, and treats patients like they would treat their own family. When you find that person, you have found the right dentist. Hold on tight, and make the best of every appointment. You and your family will enjoy the ride, rather than dreading every dentist appointment as you likely do now.

Pay attention from the start to see how well you are treated not only from the dentist, but everyone in their office. The entire team should be on board with being committed to providing exceptional care to each and every patient. Even when you make the first phone call to inquire about setting up an appointment or to ask questions regarding their services, you should feel it that they are a great place. If, on the other hand, you place that call and they seem aloof, as if they don't care if you become a patient, they are not eager to get you into their office, and the kindness doesn't come through, see it as a red flag. We want better than just having expectations met or being just OK. Anyone can be just OK, but someone who meets that standard will never be the best possible dentist for you and your family. You and your family deserve much better than just OK. In fact, the health of your mouth and overall health are depending on it being better than just OK.

The team in a highly successful dentist's office will also be top notch. The dentist will know the value of an exceptional team and will invest in them. They will know what the goals are, what is expected of them in terms of customer service, and they will have had the proper training in order to provide exemplary service. Only highly successful dentists realize this, and will make the effort to create a stellar team and office atmosphere.

Additional Exceptional Qualities

The commitment to excellent patient care and going above and beyond for everyone in the chair are not the only qualities that make for a highly successful dentist. That's certainly a big piece of the puzzle of what makes someone highly successful, but there are additional exceptional qualities you can look for. Some of the common personality traits of a highly successful dentist include:

- Being easy to talk to and being a good listener. A dentist needs to help put people at ease and calm fears and anxiety. They can easily do this through the things they say to help the patient. They can also do this by thoroughly answering questions and explaining in detail what the patient can expect. They should have no problems with working closely with others. As you realize, a dentist has to work in close contact with their patients. If someone is uncomfortable with that, it will make it difficult for them to be a great dentist. They will continuously be worried about pulling back and having more space away from the person.
- A sense of trustworthiness. Patients need to learn to trust their dentist in order to have a great relationship. The best way that this is done is through honest and open communication where the dentist takes the patient's needs and concerns into account and helps them work through each one. It may take patience to work with each patient, but the dentist who has it and demonstrates it will help build trust.
- Someone who is a passionate about what they do. They didn't go into the profession to get rich, because unless their heart and soul are in it they likely never will. Only those dentists who are truly passionate about what they do and about helping people achieve their dental goals will become highly successful. A dentist who is excited about the field will continue to keep up on new trends, technology, and will want to continue furthering their skills and knowledge, so that it can be put to good use helping their patients.
- A highly successful dentist must be a great communicator and effective leader. Not just with each patient, but with everyone they come in contact with. A dental office can only be highly successful if the dentist has a great team working in the office who can

effectively carry out the mission. Often times, it is the team of professionals at the dentist's office that you will be spending some time with, and each one needs to help reassure you that they value you as a patient. They also need to be great at communication, so they can help you with appointments, concerns, billing, etc. It takes a team of great people to help create a highly successful dentist. The dentist can't do it all on their own.

- Someone who is detailed-oriented and organized. Dental procedures often require a lot of steps and deal with small items. It's imperative that the dentist be detailed oriented in order to get it right.
- A highly successful dentist must have a sense of caring about their patients. They cannot be so absorbed in the work that they forget to ask the patient how they are doing or ask if they need a break. Showing that they care about the patient speaks volumes about their sense of compassion and understanding and will go a long way toward helping patients to feel comfortable.
- It also helps for a dentist to have some artistic skills. After all, they are helping to create a beautiful smile, so being able to master certain techniques to help them do that is a highly desirable attribute.

Chances are, you never thought much about what qualities may be needed to be a highly successful dentist. But each of these listed above play an important role in helping to give you an exceptional dental experience. Without them, you would notice and you would not be happy or completely satisfied as a patient. With them, you will feel like you have finally found the best possible dentist for you and you will not believe what an awesome difference it will make in your life and in your oral health.

More Highly Successful Qualities

There are some additional things you can look for that will help set the highly successful dentists apart. Some of these things include teaching other dentists, such as at conferences, college courses, or through continuing education. Not only do highly successful dentists continue to keep learning all the latest in the field, but they share it with others.

Highly successful dentists will also be published. They will have most likely have articles and books that they have published, offering information to the masses. They will have been quoted in articles put out by others, demonstrating their commitment to the community and the faith the journalists have in their skills and abilities.

Some of the other things that highly successful dentists do are give back to their community, and be an active part of it. They host events so that they can help the community come together and celebrate, have fun, and be a part of something. They also help those less fortunate in a variety of ways. Whether helping to support something that is going on at a local school or making mission trips to provide free dental care to those in third world countries.

In addition to being highly skilled and educated, there are many interpersonal and community-related skills and experiences that come together to make for a highly successful dentist. The dentists who stand out, rise above, and reach the highest levels of success are well-rounded individuals who are surrounded by an amazing team. They are well respected by their peers, have patients who are fiercely loyal, and will always go above and beyond for every one of their patients.

The best and most successful dentists out there cover all bases. They know how to be an effective leader to their team, they know how to prioritize their business, and they are committed to integrity in their business. They plan for success, achieve it, and continue to move the line of what they will achieve next. They stay hungry for wanting to do more in their field and help as many patients as possible.

Being highly successful is a combination of hard work, dedication to the field, a commitment to excellence, learning from setbacks, and perseverance. There isn't one description that can be given for what a highly successful dentist is, because it's a combination of things. Skills, education, teaching others, and going above and beyond are all things that are necessary, but they need to be combined with the best personality characteristics in order for the dentist to make a connection with the people. Someone can be very successful on paper, for example, and yet lack in the social skills department, which makes their patients not feel comfortable or informed.

It's important to choose a highly successful dentist. It's part of choosing the best possible dentist for you and your family. They are out there, believe me. You probably just weren't sure what to look for before. Now you have a better sense of what to look for in terms of success. Look beyond the signs and ads and see what the dentist has done and how the person treats those around them and how they fit in with the community.

CHAPTER 14

What Can I Expect at the Initial Consultation and Exam?

The moment you step into the dentist's office, you know just how important it was that you took the time to find the right one for you and your family. The energy in the office atmosphere will usually tell you a lot. It can either put you at ease or scare the daylights out of you. The last thing you want is to step into that office only to find yourself nervously waiting for your name to be called. Worse yet, you don't want to be choked up and start getting those little beads of perspiration once you do get called and make your way back to the exam room.

Taking the time to find the best possible dentist is going to help eliminate the fears and put you at ease. You will no longer cringe at the thought of having an appointment. Nor will you sit there biting your nails as you wait for your name to be called. No, once you have found the right dentist you will relax, unwind, and find ways to enjoy spending those few minutes in the waiting area. Whether flipping through a magazine or reading a few pages in the book you are currently reading, you will have no more worries at the thought of your appointments.

Your initial consultation and exam is going to create the foundation for the relationship you have with that dentist office. First impressions are a big, big deal.

Many people wonder what to expect when they go for their initial consultation and exam. Fair enough. The more you know what to expect, the less anxiety you will feel as the clock moves closer to your appointment time. Being prepared for what is going to take place helps put people at ease. While it may be helpful for you, it's also a good idea to speak with children about what to expect, to help eliminate their fears. We'll get to that a little later in this chapter, so you have an idea of what to say to get them off to a great start with the dentist.

Your First Appointment
Once you have done the necessary research and evaluation in order to find what you believe is going to be the best dentist for you and your family, it's time to make the first appointment. While the process may vary somewhat at each dental office, there are some standard things

that should take place at your first consultation and exam. Here's a breakdown of those things so you have an idea of what to expect should take place.

1. **Greeting.** The first thing that should happen when you arrive is that you should be properly greeted. Everyone who works in the dentist's office should be well trained and know how to treat every patient. Since they are expecting you, they should have things prepared and be ready for you when you arrive. You will have some paperwork to complete so that they have your contact information and some medical history. Many times they will offer those papers to you over the phone when you make the appointment. If they email them to you or tell you where to find them on their website to download and print them off, you can show up for the appointment with them already filled out. Many people find this a more convenient way to get the paperwork done, rather than trying to get it done on the spot when they show up for the appointment. The paperwork they ask you to fill out is typically required by law and is a standard procedure across practices.

2. **X-rays.** Your initial exam is going to usually include X-rays, unless there are issues that would prevent them, such as your age or diseases. Those who are pregnant are also usually excluded from getting X-rays, unless there is an emergency situation making it necessary to have them. By getting X-rays of the mouth and jawbones, the dentist can often find issues that cannot be detected with the naked eye. X-rays are helpful for helping to diagnose such conditions as cysts, tumors, impacted teeth, jawbone damage, and decay that has taken place in between teeth.

    During the first appointment, the dentist will often take a series of X-rays, including a panoramic one, which will give the dentist a good view of both the upper and lower jaw on one film. This type of X-ray is helpful because it shows your bite and how your teeth fit together. The dentist will usually show you the X-rays and go over them with you, pointing out any issues that are of concern.

4. **Examination.** Your dentist will conduct a full examination of your mouth. They will be looking at the teeth and gums, and also any specific areas of concern that have been identified by the X-rays or that you have mentioned. The dentist may identify problems or areas of concern even though you may not be aware of them yet.

The goal of every dentist is to find the problems early on, so they can be addressed and they can help keep them from becoming bigger problems later on. The sooner you treat issues, the better off you will be. Dental problems don't tend to go away, they usually start small and continue to worsen over time. The worse they get, the bigger procedure it usually is to address them, and they can go on to negatively impact other teeth, gums, or your jawbone.

5. **Cleaning.** Your initial dentist visit will usually also include a thorough cleaning with the hygienist or with the dentist. They will use special instruments to remove any build-up of plaque on or in between the teeth, scrape below the gumline, and they will usually floss and polish your teeth. During this cleaning they will usually evaluate the health of your gums. This is usually a painless process. The test they use to check the health of your gums is called a periodontal chart. They determine the health of your gums, which correlates with the numbers on the periodontal chart by measuring in millimeters (mm) the depth of the cuff of gum tissue that surrounds each tooth. As they check this, you will usually hear the person doing the evaluation saying numbers as another person records each one. The lower the number for each tooth, the better the health of that gum area is. For example, if a tooth has a 0-3 mm space without bleeding, then there are no issues and it's a healthy gum. A 3-5 mm with bleeding, on the other hand, is considered early to moderate gum disease, or the beginning of periodontitis. Those teeth with a 7mm and above rating are considered to have advanced periodontal disease and aggressive treatment will be needed. It's important to keep in mind that healthy gums do not bleed, so if yours are bleeding during the cleaning, exam, or even when you are brushing and flossing at home, there is an issue that needs to be treated.

    During the initial appointment, your dentist should evaluate for this and if there is a problem will discuss treatment options with you.

At some dentist's offices, the office manager will sit down with you to go over things. This usually comes after having your exam and cleaning. This is the time that they will discuss such issues as insurance and pricing with you. Be sure to ask questions you may have, including those about payment options. The office manager will be able to discuss the variety of options that are available for payment for the treatment that you may need. They can also answer insurance-related questions.

Once your dentist has been able to review the X-rays and to examine your mouth, they will know if there are issues of concern. If there are problems identified, such as issues with the gums, cavities, or other areas of concern, your dentist will likely recommend treatment options to you. They should be thorough in providing you with the information you need regarding what the treatment involves, how long it takes, and what you can expect from the outcome. Be sure to ask any questions you may have. A great dentist will answer all of your questions and want you to be comfortable knowing exactly what is going on and what to expect.

If you have issues that need to be addressed, and especially if you have multiple ones, your dentist will create a treatment plan for you. This will give you an idea of all of the things you need done, as well as the costs associated with them. There may be pressing issues that need to be handled right away, because they are bothering you, and there may be ones that you may be able to plan out down the line. Having a treatment plan will help get you on the right course to having the work done that you need in order to have a healthy mouth. You should be given a copy of your treatment plan to take home with you. This helps keep you informed, so that you know exactly what you need done and the costs associated with each treatment. If you are not given a treatment plan to take home, be sure to ask for a copy.

If you need treatment for a condition, they will usually make a follow-up appointment for that. If they have the time and it's a quick procedure, it may be something they can do right then. At this point you will make your appointment for the treatment, or if there were no issues you will make your next routine appointment. For those who don't have problems or concerns, you will typically have an appointment every four to six months. Once per year, you will have the X-rays and meet with the dentist for an exam, while on the other appointments you may only meet with the hygienist for a cleaning.
It's always better to address dental issues right away. Waiting to have them looked at or treated usually leads to them getting worse.
At your six-month checkup, you may only see the hygienist for a cleaning if you didn't have any areas of concern during the last appointment. However, your hygienist should ask you if you have had any problems, pain, or concerns. If you have, share them with the hygienist, who will pass that info on to the dentist. If there have been concerns,

the dentist should come in and take a look and further evaluate the situation. You also should not wait until your next six-month appointment if you have problems in between appointments. If there are problems that arise, whether it is a hurting tooth, bleeding gums, or something else, give the dentist a call and have it evaluated and addressed right away.

Many people have questions that they would love to ask their dentist or hygienist, or even the front office staff, yet they shy away from it. Don't take those questions home with you. Always ask the questions you have on your mind. I can tell you that in my office we have never minded answering questions. In fact, we want to. We want every one of our patients to feel comfortable asking questions, we want them to feel well informed, and we never want them to walk out of our office wishing they could have asked us something. Speak up, let us know, ask us, find out.

That's what we are there for, and we can't give you the info you need if you don't take the time to tell us what is on your mind or what you may be concerned with.

First Appointments Matter

Your first appointment at a new dentist's office is a big deal. You know it and so does the dentist. You may have done all your evaluating and researching to find the best possible dentist, but it's that first appointment that tells you if your assessment was correct. That one appointment should help put you at ease and let you know that you made the right choice. If it doesn't, then there is a good chance you didn't do a thorough job of evaluating and choosing an office.

Your first dental appointment is a great time to start a new chapter in your dental life. This is a time for you to create a new relationship with the dentist, regardless of what your past experiences have been like. Go into it with a positive energy, knowing that you have done the research necessary to find a great one. Trust the work you did and the pick you made. With the right dentist, you will find that you actually don't mind going in for your appointments and that your teeth look better than ever.

Your dentist is your partner in helping to keep your teeth looking great and your oral health in good condition. With the right dentist, you will feel that right from the start. They are on your side, have your best interests in mind, and are ready to serve you and meet your needs.

CHAPTER 15

Why I Am Your Dentist.

Being passionate about the dental field, I take pride in being able to help people achieve great oral health and to have an amazing smile. When my patients are happy and have something to smile about in regard to their teeth, then I feel the same way. My success is tied to how they feel about the service and care that they are receiving from my office, so we go way above and beyond to provide the best possible care around.

What Sets My Office Apart

Think back to all of the major things I have recommended to you in this book that your perfect dentist should have. Those things are all qualities that you will find in my office. Throughout the pages of this book, I have given you the tools, tips, and insider information you need so that you know what to look for when finding your best dentist. The information I have laid out in this book not only helped give you the confidence to evaluate and find the best possible dentist for you and your family, but it also put a spotlight on the reason it's so important for you to do so in the first place.

Finding the right dentist, as you know by now, is not a matter to be taken lightly.

I've explained why your smile is so important, and what happens when you don't have a great smile or you have poor oral hygiene. I've also shared why a great smile is more than just a cosmetic issue, and why just any dentist will not do. It's imperative that you have the right dentist so that you will gain the most benefits. Your dental health is too important to gamble with.

In the pages of this book, I have advised that you choose a dentist who:

- Goes above and beyond for their patients and is grateful for every one of them.
- Has a well-trained team that knows exactly how to treat patients and why it's so important to make them a priority.

- Is highly successful and is a part of their community.
- Will take the time to answer all of your questions completely, explain treatments thoroughly, and be a good listener.
- Readily offers information about payment options, so that you can find a comfortable way to pay for the treatment that you and your family are in need of.
- Has a great reputation and is well-established in the field.
- Spends time both continuing to learn about advancements in the field and teaching them to other doctors and dental health professionals.
- Gives some of their time or resources to charity to help make the world a better place.

All of these things describe me and my practice. Not only am I an award-winning dental professional, but I also have an amazing team that has been well-trained and they understand the mission of carrying out my passion for providing excellence in dental care. At my offices, we always aim to go above and beyond, because just meeting expectations of our patients is not acceptable. We want to know every patient by name, who their favorite sports team is, and what they are passionate about. In other words, we care about the person and not just their mouth.

When you have your list of all the things you are looking for in the best dentist, you can easily check them off when you consider me and my practice. We know exactly what it takes to have a great practice and we go out of our way to make it happen. We stop at nothing short of striving to be the best in order to exceed expectations. Most of our new patients come by word-of-mouth, from others who speak so highly of our office. But I wouldn't want you to merely take someone else's word for it. As laid out in this book, I would want you to take the time to fully research and evaluate my office. I'm completely comfortable with you doing that, because I know without a doubt that we will come out ahead and pass every test with flying colors.

I know firsthand how life-changing great dental care can be. I've not only lived it myself, and seen what my family members did for people, but I have seen the transformation that I've helped thousands of patients make. Having the right dentist can be a truly life-changing event. I've seen many people experience a surge in confidence following treatment. I've also seen people find the love of their life after the surge in confidence from having great teeth, as well as seen people get wonderful jobs.

Great things happen when you no longer feel you need to hide your smile or keep your mouth closed. When people feel great about their teeth, they will tend to smile more, be more outgoing, and the benefits and rewards of living like that just roll right in. Not only have I personally seen the vast life-changing differences that great treatment can give people, but I've heard the feedback, too. People often write or tell me about how their life changed following treatment in my office. Their great feedback puts a smile on my face and warms my heart, because it's exactly why we do what we do in our office.

The thorough initial exam that I explained in the prior chapter is what you can expect in my office. We are grateful for every new patient we get and we want to ensure that they are with us for a long time. We give them a thorough exam so that we can find any areas of concern and create a successful treatment plan for each and every patient. When it comes to being up front with the information and answering questions, we are dedicated to making sure you are comfortable and know exactly what your options are and what to expect. There are no surprises when it comes to the treatment that we are providing.

Why Choose Us?

We literally wrote the book on what you should look for in an excellent dentist. You are holding it in your hand. Knowing what it takes to be the best and what you should want out of a dentist, we are committed to providing you with exactly that. Our office is comprised of a team of top-notch dental professionals who believe in what they do and are passionate about doing it well. From the first phone call to set up an appointment, you will be treated with the upmost respect. We try to meet your schedule and needs and always listen to the concerns you may have, so that everything can be addressed to your satisfaction.

We are your dentist, because we know exactly what you need in a great dentist and promise to provide it. Without our loyal list of patients, we don't have a practice. We have many happy patients and that is certainly not by accident or chance. We have earned every one of them through our commitment to them and the field. Our patients trust us to provide them with honest assessments, outstanding patient services, and excellent treatments. And that's what we aim to deliver to each and every patient who walks through our doors.

Whether you just need routine cleanings and exams or you would like to explore cosmetic dentistry options, we are able to handle all of your needs. Our team has done thousands of cosmetic dentistry procedures, including porcelain veneers, tooth whitening, tooth-colored fillings, porcelain fixed bridges, porcelain crowns, bonding, and braces. We are experts in the field, keep up on the latest technologies that will help improve treatments, and provide them with an unmatched professionalism.

If you are considering sedation dentistry, we are also happy to discuss those options with you. We always maintain keeping your best interest in mind and will discuss the variety options available to you and which ones we believe you are best suited for. We also have plenty of experience when it comes to tackling that ugly matter of money. We know that not everyone has a bank account big enough to write a check for all of the treatment that they may need. Our staff is ready with the payment option information that you need, to help make it easier for you to address your oral health and have the smile you dream of.

Whether it is evaluating your current insurance, finding other plans that suit your needs, or providing payment option arrangements to consider, we are ready to help you every step of the way.

A crucial thing to remember about why I am your dentist is that I guarantee you will be happy. At our office, we always stand behind our work. If you are not happy with the treatment you have received, then we are not happy either, and we want everyone to be happy. While others may shy away from guaranteeing their work, we never do. We will always work tirelessly to ensure that are happy with the outcome of the treatments you receive. We wouldn't feel good about what we do if you walked out the door unhappy or dissatisfied with the outcome. Only when you are completely happy are we also happy. We will always stand behind our work.

We not only want you as a patient, but we care about you as a person. We want to make sure your oral health needs are met and that you love your smile. We want you to be comfortable and confident. Our mission is to be accessible to your needs. A great smile is more than just a cosmetic issue, as you have learned throughout the pages of this book. Your smile, whether good or not so good, impacts many areas of your life. We know that, so we make every effort to help you be the best version of yourself.

We know the science behind a smile, and we know the bullying, suicide, and poor grades that come from not loving the one you have. Not having a nice smile can impact both children and adults, and it's an issue we are passionate about. We want to help everyone have a great smile so they can live a better quality of life and be confident enough to chase their dreams.

Not Just Any Dentist

In an earlier chapter, I urged you to not settle for just any old dentist. Resist the urge to make it easy by choosing the one who is closest to your house, who your friend goes to, or whose name showed up first in doing an online search. That is not enough criteria for you to choose a dentist. That's essentially throwing a dart at the wall and wherever it lands, that is who will be your dentist. You can do better than that, and you owe it to yourself to do better.

I know exactly what it takes to be an excellent dentist. My skills, experience, and passion for the field takes me out of the equation of being just any old dentist. I continue to learn new technologies in the field, I teach it to others through classes and seminars, and I practice what I preach. I have thousands of patients who I have helped over the years. All of this has helped me become an award-winning dental professional. We start with a great first impression and it never diminishes from there. We believe in giving you patients the same great care that we would give to our own family members. After all, we see our team and patients as one big family.

Finally, I'd like to remind you how important personality is when choosing a dentist. Having a dentist you trust, can speak with, and feel comfortable with is huge. I mean huge. Given the opportunity, I am confident you will feel right at home in my office. I invite you to stop by my office and take a tour, meet the team, and see if you think we will be a great fit to be your next dentist.

If you find for some reason that we are not, maybe due to where you live, then I hope the information in this book will be helpful in finding the right dentist for you and your family. Whether my patient or not, I want you to have a dentist you love and teeth you feel confident and healthy with. I've laid out all of the information in this book that you need to find an awesome dentist who will be perfect for you and your family. Taking the time to do the research and evaluate will be time well-spent.

My hope is that you finish this book feeling more confident about the importance of having a great dentist, what goes into finding one, and the steps you need to take in order make it happen. If you now feel more confident in being able to find a great dentist, then this book has served its intended purpose. I believe it would be a wonderful thing if everyone found the right dentist for them, and I'm happy to give people the blueprint to help make that happen.

I'm passionate about a great smile and helping others to have one. I have come to absolute conviction on this point: A person is either going through life smiling with confidence or hiding their smile with humiliation. We all make the decision which one we will have, and need to choose wisely. There's an old Chinese proverb that says "Use your smile to change the world; don't let the world change your smile." Your smile truly can be that powerful, and when you have the right dentist you can absolutely use your smile to change the world. We can help you have that powerful smile that you want and need.

THE NEXT STEP:
Your Customized Smile Analysis

When you are ready, I urge you to schedule your **Customized Smile Analysis**, with a complimentary consultation; safe, digital x-rays (a $249 value) and exam; and report —*all without cost or obligation.*

Call us at 760-621-8700 or go to www.drmcelroy.com to schedule your own Customized Smile Analysis.

ABOUT THE AUTHOR

Dr. Gregory McElroy is a leading authority in dental implant surgery in Encinitas, CA. He has been changing lives for over 25 years. Dr. McElroy's unparalleled position as a national dental authority is the result of numerous factors, including the following:

- Bestowed the status of Diplomat from the International Dental Implant Association (Their highest level of achievement awarded.)

- Placed among the top 1% of dentists with an authority in IV Oral Conscious Sedation

- One of the first to become certified in IV Oral Conscious Sedation

- Has trained over 200 dentists throughout his career

- Has managed over 25 dental offices in California and Arizona

- Has owned and operated three dental practices in San Diego County

- Trusted industry leader.

Dr. McElroy graduated from California State University Fullerton with a degree in Biology, and he earned his Doctor of Dental Surgery degree at Georgetown University in Washington, DC.

Aside from being one of the most trusted authorities in the industry, he possesses one of the most caring souls, believing wholeheartedly in giving back through charity and community service. Committed to improving lives around the globe, he plays an active, hands-on role in all sorts of charity work.

Dr. McElroy and his team participate annually in Dentistry from The Heart, which provides free dental services to anyone in need in the local community. Dr. McElroy also donates regularly to the Wounded Warrior Project and sponsors local sports teams. The office participates in at least one full day per year of charity events which are open to the public. They generally rotate between Dentistry from The Heart, which is open to all and Smiles For Freedom which is held around Veterans Day and is focused on veterans, members of the armed forces and first responders.

Made in the USA
Columbia, SC
18 April 2021